BUREAUCRATYRANNOHYPOXIA

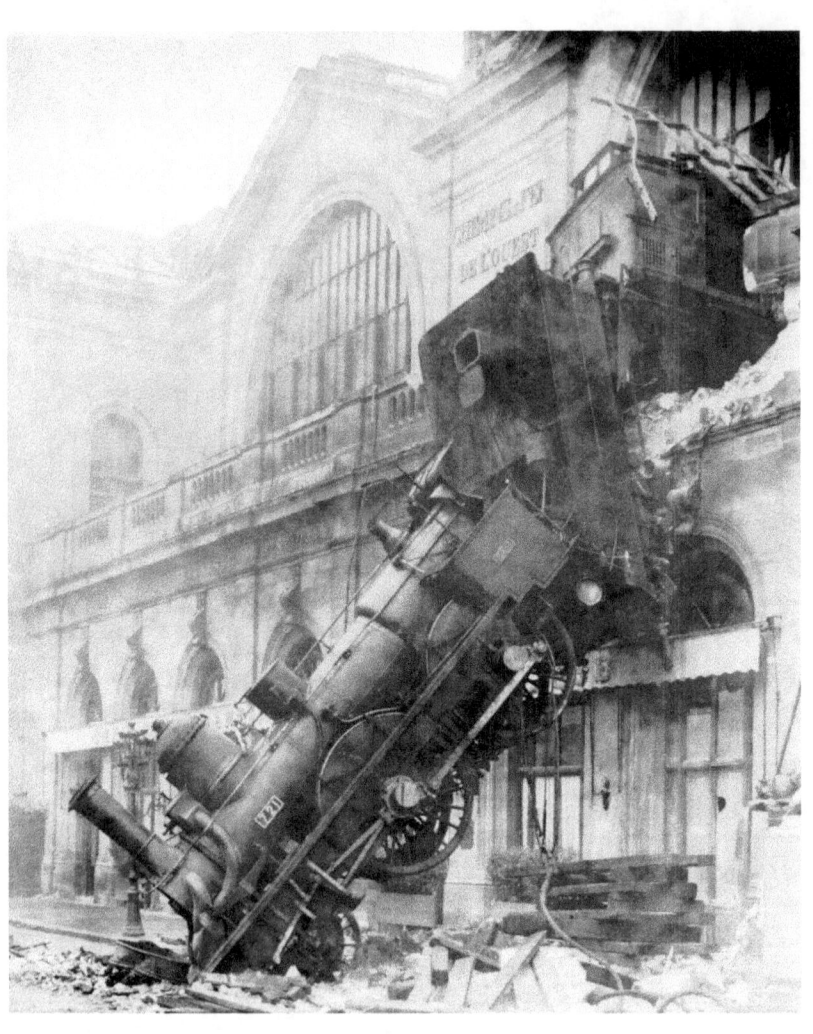

BUREAUCRATYRANNOHYPOXIA

The struggle for personal meaning

in healthcare

Letters and submissions 2010-2014

Volume 3:
If you want good personal Healthcare
See a Vet

DAVID ZIGMOND

First published 2015 by New Gnosis Publications

Printed by CreateSpace

ISBN-13: 978-1515087410
ISBN-10: 1515087417

Contents

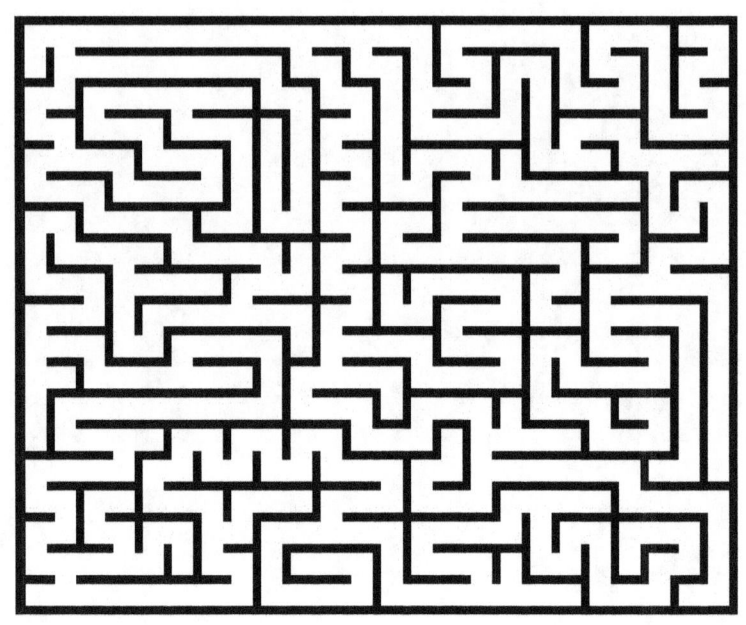

Introduction

Bureaucratyrannohypoxia is a playful neologism for my struggle with and against a new generation of tangled follies: those we have introduced into our systematised healthcare. Some of this is documented in the following collection of letters and submissions. It is the third volume in a series that explores the rich roots, but now ill fate, of pastoral healthcare: personal interactions that may foster healing and meaning. Each volume can easily be read separately, in any order. The complete anthology is known as *If You Want Good Personal Healthcare, See a Vet*. Volume One offers further historical and introductory comment for the whole series, Volume Two compiles more recent articles.

My experience has been both generated by, and anchored to, my very long tenures in both a small General Practice and as a psychiatrist in a very large hospital. These have given me equally long views of styles of management and practice, and then the fates of individuals and institutions. The nature of my observations and notions has relevance, I believe, far beyond my base of now mistrustful and mistrusted NHS Trusts.

Why and how we should care for one another is the primal question for our human welfare. Yet how we answer this becomes progressively more difficult. Certainly, massive technological advances have rendered equivalent improvements in procedural treatments. But, unintentionally, this is often at the expense of other kinds of holistic and pastoral care: those that must be rooted in personal resonance, imagination and understanding. Consequently our current healthcare culture has become increasingly scanner-sighted, but humankind-blind.

I have attempted to be part of a correcting counter-culture by many conversations and writings. This volume collects some of my letters and submissions to senior colleagues, managers, politicians and newspapers. There is a consequent great variation in length: letters to newspapers are necessarily pithy and skeletal; the submission to the Secretary of State, *Five Executive Follies,* is a long descriptive and analytical discourse on the serious unintended consequences to our healthcare of applying the 3Cs: Competition, Commissioning and Commodification.

It is difficult to gauge the effects – if any – such efforts have on executives and politicians as their survival often depends both on camouflage and remaining close to their Emergency Exits. Their responses are often diplomatically mollifying, palliating and ambiguous:

'The Minister notes your concerns with great interest. He wishes to assure you that this government is committed to providing the best personal healthcare to all who need it, at all times. The incumbent legislation (Health and Social Care Act, 2012) is now in its likely final form and further changes are deemed to be unnecessary. The Minister is confident that the new Act will drive up standards, and therefore improve the kind of care you are so rightly concerned about.'

These were the careful words of a Minister's emissary three years ago. I found him to be likeable, courteous and a good listener, but I sensed he was sent to tranquillise me. The Minister's emissary was an exceptional and privileged response for me: his message was not. So far, events are proving him wrong.

Such scenarios are, of course, part of a much larger whole. But the technical details often make the links inscrutable to an outsider. To help the perplexed reader place the parochial within the global, I have included a critical Glossary.

David Zigmond, August 2015

Glossary of Institutional Terms

Much of the writing of this Volume encounters our increasing and severe healthcare conundra: these are largely consequent to our over-industrialisation of the Medical Model. This has become particularly clear in the cultural and political turmoil besetting Britain's National Health Service.

The interest and importance of these issues extends far beyond this already vast arena, but the organisational events are very complex and often difficult to understand: examples may need explanation. This is even more likely for readers who are not healthcare workers or British residents.

As a bridge to clarity and comprehension, I have constructed this critical glossary of key terms. Many of the italicised words are cross-referenced: this helps to give an outline of the current System's skeleton. Some key terms are worth highlighting but are widely known and understood: for economy of space I have italicised but not glossaried these.

Algorithm. A templated and flow-charted system of defined and logical steps prescribed to analyse and manage identified problems. Can be readily diagrammed and computerised. Has rapid appeal due to its standardised reproducibility, apparent clarity, precision and logic. Disadvantages: deals poorly with real-life's ambiguity, variation, meaning and complexity. Can displace individually responsive and intelligent judgement and imagination.

Appraisals for healthcare staff. A formal procedure whose purpose is to monitor and assure quality and safety of professional performance and development. Much effort has been made to standardise and, when possible, quantify such complex evaluations. Guidance has been sought from the newer professions of business management and consultancy. The aspiration is far less controvertible than the results: for the formalistic segues easily to the formulaic. Subsequent attempts to make procedure 'fair and comprehensive' commonly become burdensome, blind and bureaucratic. Generally professionals have described their experiences of appraisals as elaborate rituals of proffered compliance and verbalised obedience. Far fewer report the kind of intelligent searching dialogue that will helpfully identify or clarify important problems.

Balint. Michael Balint (1896-1970) was a psychoanalyst who, in the 1950s and 1960s, explored the 'subtext' of medical consultations. He started with a small group of London GPs, but his influence expanded to galvanise a generation of doctors to think about inexplicit meaning, encoded actions and attachments, and the possibility of both treatment and illness as kinds of preverbal or paraverbal language. Many GPs experienced their work as enriched and enlightened by such informal and qualitative research. This brief, rich flowering was largely extinguished by the rapid rise of systems that demanded quantification, standardised codes, and mass-reproducibility.

Evidence Based Medicine has great difficulty accommodating Balint's subtle invitations to explore meaning.

Care Quality Commission (CQC*).* A governmental network of healthcare inspectors. This is similar in mission to the *Appraisal* of professional individuals, but applied to the healthcare organisation that employs them. As with Appraisals, the task is certainly necessary and important but its sensible and accurate execution very difficult. Again, presentations of formulaic compliance can easily mask deeper lack of integrity. The shocking debacle at *Mid Staffs* examples what can be missed by 'competent' yet routinised methods of inspection.

Clinical Commissioning Group (CCG). A recently mandated executive network for deciding, defining, procuring and purchasing the healthcare needs of an allocated geographical population. The boards are now dominated by local GPs but contain other healthcare professionals and lay members. The CCG has replaced the *Primary Care Trust (PCT)*, which was administered, ultimately, by non-clinical managers.

The aspiration – for democratic healthcare decisions that are locally responsive and responsible, and professionally decided – seems laudable. The unravelling reality is less so: multitasking, overmanaged and weary GPs already have much diminished time for their traditional role as personal physicians and cannot give adequate, good attention to this new and very complex task. The result is an expedient short-circuiting to a hastily assembled (and thus often not competent) network of oligarchies that are themselves likely to be in thrall to a very flawed *Internal Market*.

Cognitive Behaviour Therapy (CBT). An attempt to schematise and standardise therapeutic psychological contact for the mentally or behaviourally troubled. It is largely based on depersonalised diagnostic categories, focused on the symptomatic and explicit, and guided by *algorithms* and *Care*

Pathways. It is readily (if speciously) computer-coded and measurable: CBT thus has appeal to planners, economists, managers and the kinds of practitioners who share their mindset. The limitations are similar to all algorithms and Care Pathways: the model has difficulty with complexity, variation, meaning and imagination – and thus can easily impoverish practitioners' personal resources to deal with these.

Commissioning. A currently common term for design, negotiation and procurement of services within the marketised NHS. Like other devices to industrialise and monetarise healthcare it is least problematic when applied to healthcare problems that are generally resolved rapidly and reliably by standardised technical procedure (eg hip replacements). *Pastoral Healthcare* (eg psychiatry) starkly exposes its limitations.

Commodification. The attempt to treat and process all healthcare activities as if they are manufactured objects or geophysical resources. This can work relatively well in tasks that have clear and stable boundaries. *Pastoral Healthcare*, by contrast, needs vocational and holistic attitudes that cannot be processed in this way. Nevertheless, commodification makes welcome sense to planners and managers in conducting many aspects of the *Internal Market*. Experiences from frontline health workers are far less tidy: for many years there have been mounting, frustrated expressions of clinical and personal meaninglessness and the stymying of good personal care.

Community Mental Health Team (CMHT). Thirty years ago CMHTs were vaunted as a progressive face of the future, consummated by the closure of the old *Mental Hospitals*. Instead mentally distressed patients would be speedily streamed to community-based specialisms. The specialists themselves professionally progress via certified trainings rather than personal qualities or vocation. Recent healthcare management thinking – much derived from 1980s Japanese car manufacturing – promised more efficient, accessible and responsive help. As elsewhere in the NHS, this attempt to industrialise pastoral healthcare produces results that often become inefficient and perverse.

Evidence-based Medicine (EBM). This has been introduced into healthcare to optimise the reliability and efficiency of therapeutic interventions. The idea is to invest in language and procedures that are officially sanctioned by scientific rigour, and then *Governance*. Healthcare economists and planners favour EBM because it is apparently objective, clear and unambiguous – and can then extirpate the errors and obfuscations of the personal and subjective. In this way *Quantification*, *Standardisation* and *Commodification* are all expedited. EBM thus becomes a key component in the *Internal Market*.

EBM is yet another example from healthcare of how a model's attractive simplicity may be woefully inadequate for complex realities. EBM has mostly operated from evidence restricted to the quantifiable and reproducible. This makes a base that is deemed 'safe', but is also narrow and rigid. It may be necessary, but it often is not sufficient. Problems arise because EBM may be loaded with an authority it cannot bear. Very often the most important aspects of human experience and variation cannot be directly measured or objectified. This is far more than any administrative anomaly: for the unmappable area is the massive – yet vulnerable – human heart of healthcare. EBM, in compatible areas, may be a valuable guiding principle: aggrandised to wider and rigid diktat, it can do real harm.

Increased Access to Psychological Treatment Services (IAPTS). A late parallel, and equivalent, to *CMHTs*. The task focus is therapeutic psychology (not psychiatry). Similar processes are used to identify, stream and manage problems: diagnoses, *Care Pathways* and (especially) the use of *CBT* as a procedural intervention. The system is designed to be easily compatible with electronic informatics, the *Internal Market* and *Payment by Results*. Some also argue that it helps equity and fairness of distribution. The flaws are largely common to those of the *CMHT*.

Internal Market. In the early 1990s this was a seminal and radical idea: to introduce monetarist values and mechanisms to nationalised healthcare. The enormous federal cooperative network would be broken up into economically and occupationally autarkic *NHS Trusts*. Wide and informal affiliations were replaced by a complex system of *Purchaser-Provider Splits*, which need tending by ceaseless negotiations to facilitate 'trade' between the Trusts. Computerised, quantifiable data, *Care Pathways* and *Payment by Results* are all necessary developments to service this Internal Market. The idea is to positively influence motivation and focus attention. After more than twenty years' evolution the results are mixed and highly contentious. Many longer-term observers (myself included) assess the losses as much greater than the gains. Since the recent Health and Social Care Act there is now more possibility of an external market: this amplifies contention.

Mid-Staffs. Refers to the Mid Staffordshire NHS Trust. In recent years perplexed and appalled attention has focused on the clear and massive failures and abuses of care uncovered in this NHS hospital. The widespread institutional human disengagement has been shocking enough. Further grotesquerie is provided by the attractive and respectable public persona of the Trust: it had received very favourable reports from routine official inspections, eg by the *CQC*. Mid Staffs is one of many egregious examples of concealed inhumanities in current NHS healthcare, though the most notorious. Many see Mid Staffs as being a kind of diabolic iconic: a harsh signal of the consequences of abandoning healthcare's primal task of human recognition and connection. Such abandonment, it is argued, is due largely to the rise of the *Internal Market's* 3Cs (Competition, Commissioning and Commodification) and a culture cowed by managed demands for numerous, rigid and narrow *targets* and *PBR*. Subsequent statements from Mid Staffs' employees have described a bullied and intimidated work culture redolent of factory workers a century earlier.

National Institute for Health and Care Excellence (NICE). A governmentally appointed network of experts tasked with evaluating and applying *EBM* in specified areas of healthcare. As its operational nucleus is EBM, it has the same assets, limitations and liabilities. Thus NICE makes its most competent contributions to healthcare problems that are clearly physically defined, and which can then be reliably resolved or contained by standardised physical procedures.

So, NICE-prescribed frameworks usually make good and useful (though not infallible) contributions to the care of, say, Diabetes or Hypertension. Yet this kind of *algorithmic* management fares far less well with the vast human variations of pastoral healthcare (eg mood disturbance or alcoholism) where individual practitioners' wisdom, experience and subtle hues of judgement are central and indispensable.

Pastoral Healthcare. A term little used, but increasingly needed. It refers to our guiding human matrix of care: all those personal influences that comfort, heal, guide, contain, encourage, vitalise and illuminate. Pastoral healthcare thus extends far beyond any procedure or formula. Although certainly including such activities as personally attuned 'mental healthcare' or 'psychotherapy', it is not confined to these. Good Pastoral Healthcare is synonymous with the heart, soul and broader intellect involved throughout our encounters with others' distress. Like so many holistic activities, its subtler enactments cannot be readily measured, coded or proceduralised: Pastoral Healthcare thus tends to be neglected, displaced or destroyed by a culture dominated by the *Internal Market* and such satellite procedures as *Payment by Results, Evidence Based Medicine, Quality Outcome Frameworks* etc.

Payment by Results (PBR). The intention and thinking behind this kind of infusion of commercial motivation is relatively clear. It often galvanises manufacturing industries. Yet the consequences – when applied to complex human welfare – become frequently obscure, tangled and perverse. Results of complex activities are often difficult to define, measure or predict. Motivation in welfare is – and should be – much broader and more complex than that of commerce. Unbridled PBR in healthcare provides specious statistics, bad science and egregiously perverse incentives.

Primary Care Trust (PCT). For several years this body preceded the *CCG* in managing the trade and conduct of Community Practitioners (GPs, Dentists, Pharmacists, District Nurses, Health Visitors, Chiropodists etc). It was managed largely by non-clinicians: the transition to CCGs brings doubtful benefits as few GPs can maintain the long-term personal resources necessary for the complexity and size of the task.

QUOF (Quality Outcomes Framework). A complex system of remuneration for GPs, constituting a kind of 'performance related pay'. This is based on electronically guided and recorded *Specific Performance Indicators,* themselves based on *algorithms* and *Care Pathways* designed by governmental think-tanks and committees. The resultant computerised systems monitor and signal how each practitioner is managing each encounter with a patient with a chronic disease or risk. QUOF has thus brought the government and the computer into the centre of the consulting room in an unprecedented way. The results are mixed. The gains are most clear in bringing more vigilant and systematic management to high risk conditions where therapeutics are clearly effective (eg Hypertension and

Coronary Heart Disease), and detection of some other areas of significant risk/poor engagement. The losses are from displacement. Computer informatics and governmentally dictated tasks replace subtle, personally nuanced exchanges that are essential for comfort, understanding and healing influences. Such undesignated 'softer' activities are also essential to NHS staff morale. The QUOF-directed GP has become more of a public health commissar than a personal physician: patients are increasingly 'efficiently' treated, but poorly understood.

Bureaucratyrannohypoxia

An open letter to
Mental Health Services Director

Dear Director of Mental Health Services

My experience with an urgent psychiatric problem: an instructive example of current institutional complexity, rigidity and unresponsiveness. Bureaucratyrannohypoxia

In a recent phone call, I described briefly a fresh episode to you. It seemed (to me) a good example of the rising tide of depersonalised, procedural complexity. This burgeoning is burdensome: obstructive to sensible, sensitive, attachment-respectful care. It is often confusing, frustrating and disheartening for professionals, patients and possibly (even) managers. It is very expensive.

Before time submerges memory, I want to record this episode, and some of my thoughts about it. The episode is one of many: I choose just one, for focus and dissection.

My detail is very deliberate: please take your time.

1. The Prelude

Early one afternoon (in June 2010) I am telephoned by the mother of a 39-year-old woman. The mother herself is clearly fearful and distressed by convergent difficulties gathering around her daughter: "Ellie is crying all the time ... she won't eat and yesterday got drunk (again) ... she was doing so well until she foolishly and briefly tried to get back together with Omar (ex-partner) ... Just one night, but she accidentally got pregnant ... She was shocked and realised it was a terrible mistake. She had a Termination, but when Omar found out, he 'went mental' with rage and broke her arm so badly she had to have complicated operations, and now cannot use it ... She can't look after her little boy (Sam, age 4), so my sister is looking after him ... Ellie says her life is so useless and painful, she'd rather not have it ... I've got a disabled husband: I can't stay with her ... She doesn't want to go into hospital, she's had bad experiences there ... Can you help us, Doctor? ..."

*

Ellie joined my GP list three months ago. I had seen her twice for routine appointments. She told me she was a 'refugee' from an acrimoniously broken relationship with Omar, and had moved across London to create both distance and defensible space. My more psychiatric questions clarified a pattern of several years' fluctuating Reactive Depression and spasmodic alcoholic consolation. She told me of her failed attempts to make a durable, loving bond with a man. Each ended with a variety of hurt, abuse, betrayal and derogation. It needed little prompting for her to talk of the developmental roots of this: her descriptions of a charismatic, powerful but sarcastic and alcoholically violent father; a cravenly collusive and melancholically abstracted mother. Her manner was naïve, warm, submissively apologetic, distressed and affecting. She was tearfully and copiously grateful for my interest in her current dilemma and its history, both recent and ancient. I realised how important quality and continuity of personal care would be for her. While re-prescribing her established anti-depressants, I communicated this to her: as her GP I offered her both periodic anchorage and guided-support across her Sea of Troubles. I talked with her of possible help from longer-term Counselling and Alcohol Services. We conjured and glimpsed future possible scenarios from a rebuilt life. She left me, both times, with a moist-eyed smile and a proffered, warm, firm handshake.

*

My urgent visit to her revealed rapid disintegration. Having retreated into her bed and nightclothes, her chaotic and spasmodic speech was rent further by anguished sobbing. Her physical needs and safety were provided by her mother, now buckling under the heavy contagion of distress. Despite the intense level of emotional disturbance, I was able to establish sufficient recognition, communication and alliance with Ellie to calm and contain them both. I held her hand, to gently push out a fragile bridge to the small island in Ellie that could think and speak clearly. We established that she was so overwhelmed by her life-events, and her distress, that she could no longer competently care for herself and would need supervised care, until recovery. I told them I would try to arrange this for her, at home. I then returned to my surgery, to record a diagnostic formulation that would be required from the Mental Health Team(s).

'Acute Severe Schizoaffective Reaction/Agitated Reactive Depression (choose either). Risk to Self only (probably undeliberate). Co-operative/motivated to help. Previous binge-drinking. Needing immediate supervised care (at home, if possible). Complex and chronic emotional/family/relationship problems: will need much reconstructive psych. work later.'

That would do.

2. Complex Times: The Institutional Response 2010

On arriving back at my surgery I ring my Community Mental Health Team for contact details and procedural advice. I am given these, and contact the Crisis Team Manager, after much delay, via a Paging Service. The eventual telephone contact is one of a unilateral pro-forma interrogation (of me), rather than any kind of colleagueial dialogue. Her questions are formulaic, and I have the sense that the questioner is guided more by institutional rules than relevant experience. At the end of her questions she tells me that a member of her Team would be able to visit at an unspecified time within the next four hours and that it is essential that I am present, for the safety of her staff. I tell her that Ellie is forlorn and passively imploded: she is a possible hazard only to herself, not imminently and only indirectly. Also this institutional safeguard takes no account of my other work: I have a busy Practice to run.

The young manager is curt and adamant: Team Policy is not negotiable. We are at an impasse: it is impossible for me to comply. I now fractiously ask if she has any ideas as to how I may get Ellie urgently cared for, at home. She brightens with a nascent possibility: if I send Ellie to St Thomas' A&E Department after 6 pm, she will be seen by the OOH Emergency Psychiatric Team there, and they will assess her, and my suggestion.

*

After 6 pm I manage to contact the Duty Psychiatrist after much searching via the Hospital Switchboard. I tell him the outline of the current crisis and some selected antecedents. He is sympathetic in manner and pragmatic in plan. I do not tell him of my freshly-exited impasse with the Crisis Team, lest this somehow invalidates my request. He cordially suggests I send Ellie to A&E, where someone from the Emergency Team will assess her. A much briefer but much more dialogic and helpful phone call, this. I express my relief and gratitude.

*

I now call Ellie: her mother answers, fatigued and expectant. I outline the plan. She responds with realistic despondency and deferral: "Ellie's now exhausted and asleep … She's in no state to go to hospital and wait around for someone to ask her lots of questions. Can I take her tomorrow, after she's had a night's sleep?" This deferral makes sense to me, though I simultaneously sense my unfair frustration with their lack of 'compliance' to The System.

I call back the hospital Duty Psychiatrist and tell him of these developments. She will arrive the next morning at A&E. I will fax a letter with some helpful background and my reasons for recommending Home Treatment, by the Emergency Team who can assess her in A&E.

No, he says. Do not send a letter as this will be received within ordinary working hours, deemed a procedurally incorrect GP referral, returned to me with the instruction to re-contact the Crisis Team and start again. However, if I get the patient and mother to attend A&E, and make no mention of all our prior communications, it would be treated as a fresh self-referral and not sent back to me. As co-conspirator, he is inventive and supportive: he knows The System. Such stealth and deceit is essential to procure what I know is necessary for Ellie. And to return home that night. It has taken me 2½ hours.

The time later taken by Staff in A&E, and later by the Home Treatment Team, merely to assess and decide, would be much longer.

3. Simpler Times: The Institutional Response 1970s-80s

From the early 1970s I have had several decades working in, and then alongside, psychiatric services (the latter as a Principal GP). The response I now describe is drawn from many similar incidents in this earlier period, in which I was either active, or witness to. It is typical of the better practice of the time. The scenario is thus a fictitious graft of those old experiences onto my more recent problem with Ellie.

*

After seeing Ellie at home, I immediately phone Dr G, the Consultant Psychiatrist at Highmount Mental Hospital. Dr G is aged about 50, and has been a consultant there for ten years. He has got to know many of the GPs on his patch and is interested in, and respectful of, the very different psychological qualities, styles and abilities that the different practitioners bring to the encounters with complex emotional distress. We have had warm and efficient problem-exchanges several times over five years. I sense he has a good sense of my human and professional strengths, deficits and (I secretly hope) vulnerabilities.

When I call Highmount I am initially put through to Linda, his secretary. She has a bright, alert and friendly manner and is clearly interested in her work. We immediately recognise the other's voice: we have a short bantering diversion, the kind of safe familiarity that keeps morale and relationships buoyant in turbulent waters. I tell Linda about my patient Ellie, in outline, and what I am hoping Dr G will arrange. She tells me that Dr G is busy on the Wards, and that he will call me in an hour.

Dr G calls me as arranged. It is calming and reassuring to hear his voice. Linda has briefly briefed him, and he invites me to tell him what else I think is most salient. His few questions are intelligently chosen, from long and wide experience. He understands a complex situation with graceful and subtle speed. My conversation with him has lasted only five minutes, but it is full and consummate.

He will get Ellie visited in the next couple of hours, he says. He's not sure who will go, either himself or his trusty, long-affiliated CPN, Patrick. Either Patrick or Dr G will call me the next morning and let me know what they have decided and implemented.

Dr G makes his expected second call to me. He had visited and spoken to Ellie and her mother for about half an hour: it was harrowing, affecting contact, and the time taken matched what he needed to know, as well as the sufferers' near-exhausted emotional resources. They had all agreed to try caring for her at home, unless she deteriorated. Patrick would visit daily, and would also liaise with Social Services. Dr G would revisit later in the week. The usual medications were specified and prescribed. Another short but full collegial dialogue: concise, companionable, accommodating, flexible and satisfying.

4. Comparisons, contrasts and comments

These different scenarios will be familiar to all older Practitioners who have retained memory and interest. Likewise, I believe, my frustrations and critique. The following brief comments are fairly random. Some problems I identify may have become insoluble: I hope I am wrong.

The old system of Consultant General Psychiatrist-managed small teams covering In-Patients, Out-Patients, Domiciliary Visiting and (even) Long-Stay wards was much more intelligently responsive, interpersonally continuous and economically-efficient. (I would accept that only better Consultant-teams from that era support my argument.)

Senior Psychiatrists in that earlier period were, when appointed, usually both more widely experienced and older than is now the case: Consultant Psychiatrists typically started their tenure aged about 40 years, having worked for many years as Physicians or General Practitioners, before turning to Psychiatry.

The equivalent today is a Practitioner almost ten years younger, with often very little medical experience. Furthermore, the psychiatric experience they have had is likely to expose them more to academic or managerial meetings, and far less to the complexities of longer-term understanding and response to individual anguish. The contemporary Consultant is thus likely to be algorithmically well-trained, but interpersonally (and Clinically) sparsely experienced and educated. This statement does not reflect the innate calibre of the practitioners, rather the consequences of the systems that train and employ them. The economics and design of training and services are now subsumed excessively to the Medical Model and a derivative Commissioning Economy. These tend to confer specious order and authority to situations poorly understood or engaged with. It is easy to understand the allure of thinking and language that seems to provide such speedy definition and clarity. In my view it usually requires considerable clinical experience to develop a subtle understanding of the limitations of the Medical Model, in order to be able to selectively and competently discard it; to make way for the more creatively empathic and imaginative aspects of growth and healing.

'Assessments' and 'Treatments' are often administered by inexperienced Multi-Disciplinary Team Practitioners, who are themselves programmed, strictured and structured by algorithms, guidelines or diktats from NICE, relevant Trusts, etc. These commissarial imperatives are themselves navigated almost entirely via the Medical Model and the Commissioning Economy.

I have an endless stream of examples of inexperienced MDT workers conducting lengthy, formulaic assessments, leaving an indigestible, long trail of bureaucracy and documentation. Amidst such dogged (sometimes zealous) compliance to The System, the patient feels exhausted, overpowered and unheard. This pattern is conveyed to me regularly. Paradoxically, the inflexible overuse of the Medical Model seems more likely with younger Clinical Psychologists, OTs, Social Workers, RMNs, etc, perhaps because they are prone to use the model anxiously and defensively. Spectres of Medical incompetence or negligence are so much easier to tame or side-step after lengthy and substantial Clinical experience. In my view these kind of Practitioners should revert to auxiliary, complementary or supportive roles in relationship to the Principal Psychiatric Practitioner ('PPP" = Consultant or Deputy) who would then be freer to 'cut to the chase'. In the previous era, when the PPP delegated to other Practitioners with skill and sensitivity, then administration and bureaucracy was light and dextrous and staff morale was much higher. People mostly did what they were good at, and felt safer and more valued.

Unanswerable questions? Impossible options? In order to reclaim and regrow some of the departing skills and wisdom (I would designate them as 'Holistic', 'Psychodynamic' or 'Humanistic'), we need to undo many recent 'advances' (which I suggest are not). Among the many conundrae, some involve training and staffing: how can we selectively undo rapid specialist training and encourage might-be psychiatrists to be immersed as (say) Physicians or GPs for several years first? Could consultant status be strengthened but delayed for several years? How could applicants happily accept this as part of an unengineered and gentle acquisition of wisdom, for the benefit of themselves, their therapeutic eco-systems, their patients? Can this possibly fit alongside the near ubiquitous streamlining and acceleration of NHS Professional career pathways? Likewise, could we dismantle current MDTs and get the non-PPP psychiatric-care workers to reclaim, and re-energise, with pride and cooperation, traditional but more limited roles, once valued but now atrophied from disuse?

No easy answers to such questions, even if desired. No Reset button.

The work of all in Public Welfare has become increasingly in thrall to doctrines and mindsets from Health and Safety, corporate, competitive industry and policing. The resulting Bureaucratyrannohypoxia has coalesced to a Culture that ensnares and suffocates us all. The fragile but rich influences of healing, humanism and holism are now almost extinguished. Likewise the better kind of confederate socialism that used to contain the NHS. How can we resuscitate and rehabilitate these?

Such questions are crucial far beyond our local responsibilities or individual career spans. I hope this open letter will provide some spark and fuel for our further thought and discussion. I look forward to both.

Ω

Dear Andrew Lansley, MP
(Secretary of State for Health 2011)

Commodification, commissioning and commercialisation: the growing threats to personal healthcare

I have been an inner city Principal GP since the 1970s and have witnessed and implemented the successive changes. All have been well intentioned, and all have had adverse unintended consequences. Changes towards commodification, commissioning and commercialisation of healthcare are particularly destructive where 'soft skills' and personal investment are crucial.

We are at the edge of another tranche of accelerated changes. In the near future I fear for the integrity of my work and the personal care of my patients. Beyond that, almost certainly, I shall become a patient: I have a dread of care by agencies and teams with no personal experience or knowledge of me, and little skills or interest to invest in these.

I enclose an analytical summary of my last few years' observation and thoughts about these very difficult and important healthcare issues. *Five Executive Follies* pursues lines of enquiry that may be unfamiliar for you, but may be rewarding. It has been written very carefully and requires similar attention to best assimilate and understand. Despite your enormous volume of written communication and other work, I hope you will find time for this.

I write to stimulate thought and creative discussion. I welcome any further contact from either you, or one of your deputies.

Thank you for your attention and interest.

Ω

Five Executive Follies

How commodification imperils compassion in personal healthcare

Summary: Commodification, competition and commercialisation are often introduced as agents of efficiency into State welfare services. In healthcare all of these may, unwittingly, lead to a loss of 'soft skills'; personal understanding and compassion. The human and economic cost is considerable. How this happens is not obvious. This article explains.

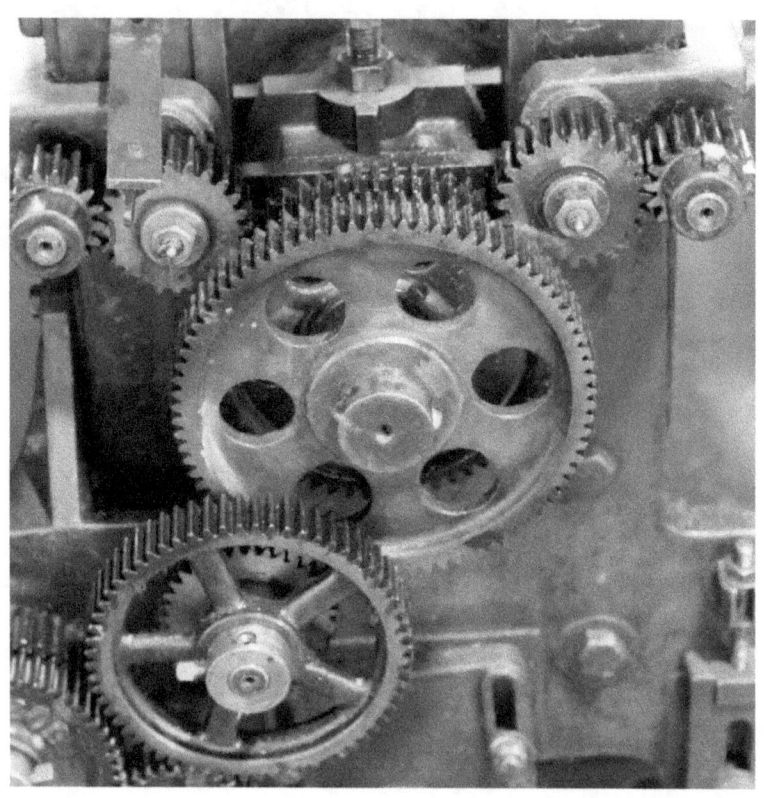

Prologue

The threat to healthcare from inadequate resources or management has become a little-challenged truism: easy to understand and demonstrate. Healthcare is now submissive to our Management Culture: a world which then authoritatively delegates all human problems to specialists and their executive actions. All this can seem simple, sensible and correct.

The reality is more complex. Paradoxically, there is an additional and opposing, though less obvious, threat to our healthcare: an *excess* of such management, specialist activities and resources – but misplaced. This more subtle and countercultural reality is – it is proposed here – responsible for much of our current system's incapacity to imaginatively address individual variation. Such obliviousness to human diversity and complexity has serious consequences. The more stark examples of failures of physical care make headlines that are hard to understand or even believe. In contrast, failures of personal understanding, and thus therapeutic and compassionate engagement, are usually born invisibly, painfully and privately. Such are the perils of abdicating our capacity to conceive or care more holistically.

Compassion becomes an inevitable casualty whenever personal attunement or engagement are compromised. The word 'compassion' derives its meaning from a Latin root 'to suffer together', thus offering a 'transpersonal' psychology; one drawing from exchanges of resonance and imagination. This is often very different from distancing, 'objective' psychologies used unilaterally by healthcare professionals to pathologise, categorise and commodify in attempts to tightly manage healthcare. Yet there are many studies showing how an empathic bond conveying compassion is a powerful source of comfort and healing for the sufferer, and work-satisfaction (and healing) for the healer.

The skilled evocation of compassion often has powerful effects, but is a subtle activity. This was well recognised and explored by previous generations of practitioners. It now ails amidst hardy slogans of 'Increased Patient Choice' and 'Ensuring quality of care is always central'. How could this cme about? The causal paradoxes and anomalies have been poorly recognised and understood. What follows dissects and explores.

*

Five Executive Follies: How commodification imperils compassion in personal healthcare

The fatal metaphor of progress, which means leaving things behind us, has utterly obscured the real idea of growth, which means leaving things inside us.
GK Chesterton, *Fancies versus Fads*, 1923

We are living longer, more complex lives. Our technological possibilities multiply. Inevitably healthcare expectations, then demands, burgeon. To manage all this, an Industrial Revolution has been unleashed in the NHS. This revolution is itself guided by a core phalanx of doctrines. These are independent of other political considerations or affiliations, and implicitly embraced by all. Such assumptions have developed from cultural changes rooted in our advanced industrialised ways of life. These predicate often unconscious values and mind-sets. Consequently, our rubric for healthcare has become increasingly of *applied sciences*, leaving *humanities* peripheral and disregarded. The tasks then become reduced to engineering tissues or behaviours, rather than extension to nurturing human understanding and contact.

The doctrines that flow from such assumed applied science and industrialisation may thus offer real help in discretion, but an added tranche of folly in excess. Like many truisms, they turn specious, then hazardous. The Law of Unintended Consequences becomes evident: industrialising healthcare, much to our perplexity, is responsible for very substantial 'collateral damage'. Despite allocating ever-increasing resources, in certain areas, our therapeutic and compassionate engagement is poorer. The progressive loss of quality and continuity of personal contact – essential elements of compassion – are crucial factors. This brief survey samples how these difficulties constellate.

37

Below are itemised these interlocking cardinal notions. Consequences of their over-use are portrayed. In the final section, authentic vignettes illustrate how these Five Executive Follies converge; what happens to our care.

Failure to accurately conceive the essential nature and limitations of the medical model is a primal difficulty. Unbridled objectification may soon turn to alienation. The underlying misconceptions unwittingly arise from 'category errors' that are very powerful, yet rarely distinguished or discussed. Such discernment requires unfamiliar thought about our working axioms. For this reason our first folly receives the lengthiest deliberation. The later appendix offers a tabulated summary and illustrative graphs.

1. Medical diagnoses and treatment models are the most effective for dealing with human ailments. These methods are clear, authoritative and evidence-based. They should be precedent wherever possible.

This is mostly and uncontentiously true when dealing with 'structural' diseases of the body, particularly where the condition is localised and acute. Common examples: hip fracture, pneumonia, appendicitis. With any of these we are grateful and satisfied with competent and courteous biomechanical attention. With other kinds of health problems this effectiveness becomes much less clear. The 'medical model' then loses its unrivalled command and precision; for example, when dealing with complaints that are not structural, but experiential, 'functional' and stress-related. What are these? They include an ocean of ill-defined but physically distressing complaints which present to GPs and various healers; they become loosely packaged with labels such as migraines, dyspepsia, dysmenorrhoea, tension headaches, IBS, PMS and ME. Then there is the vast range of human anguish – the psychiatrically classified Mental Disorders: disturbances of behaviour, appetite, mood or impulse (BAMI).

There is a useful general equation that can guide our designation and understanding:

structural change = disease; functional disorder = dis-ease.

Although the words look very similar, our optimal methods for approaching and apprehending them often need to be very different. For example: structural disease can be tightly clustered into *generic* diagnoses where individual variation and meaning are relatively unimportant. 'One size fits all.' In contrast, functional dis-ease is more likely to be *idiomorphic*: the generic pattern now less decisive, but the individual meaning and variation crucial. 'Only the wearer knows where the shoe pinches.' As we will see, erroneous conflation of the two leads to many other follies in practice, from individual consultations to national healthcare planning. Such conflation is easily done, and then often very hard to undo. Because of its importance, this subtle but powerful distinction is worth paying time and attention to understand

The dazzling success of biomedical science in tackling many structural diseases may blind our perception of its competent boundaries. Dazzled, we fail to see that overuse of medical diagnosis and treatment in areas of dis-ease becomes counter-productive. This kind of misplacement is complexly inefficient: it frequently leads to eclipse or displacement of more personal and fruitful types of dialogue and understanding – the keys to healing, growth and resolution. Without these, compassion perishes.

There are problems, too, about the integrity, the 'realness', of our research and knowledge when we confuse or conflate these two territories, of disease and dis-ease. Current currencies of quantification and 'evidence-basis' are now a shibboleth to any 'service provision'. Despite this assigned pre-eminence, such esteemed quantitative research becomes less valid when applied away from the shoreline of solid-state pathology: disease. Problems arise when investigating dis-ease because this is primarily a form of communicated experience, not a stable or simple physical state. Yet, no inner experience can be measured directly. We can only access and measure external, associated behaviours or verbal reports. This is hard for those healthcare workers in thrall to objective scientific method: they hope and believe that their measurements or observations reliably indicate private experience. But such formulated indices are, alas, never equations. Research of internal experience here becomes inescapably 'contaminated' by a myriad of personal, relational or institutional factors. For example, attempts to measure 'mood' or 'well-being' are fraught with subjective and interpersonal intrusions and distortions and can never match the clarity or precision of, say, blood electrolytes. To compound the problem, the contaminating factors (eg of conscious or unconscious suggestion, influence or wish) are themselves unmeasurable. In this welter of uncertainties, away from bodily structural disease, science can only operate with severely annotated compromises: 'pscience'. Organisationally and economically, this introduces myriad tangles to the meaning and integrity of statistics. projects such as 'Commissioning' and 'Payment by Results' then entice specious clarity, with all its inevitable difficulties and corruptions.

All cultures are defined by a prevailing rhetoric. In our industrialised healthcare the categorised and the quantified are now hegemonic. Flawed pscience is now precedent to an unquantified vernacular, however apposite. Such staticised pscience thus proceeds with a kind of abstracted, regal authority in areas of delicate interpersonal uncertainty. This is a growing problem, most clearly in psychiatry and primary care: here the insidious change has become cultural, and has, by definition, led to a diminution of professional awareness, analysis and debate. The interpersonal skills deriving from these perish, too.

Such areas of healthcare need to reclaim those receding and very different kinds of imaginative intelligence. For example, pscience is likely to assess a distressed person by administering a quantifiable mood questionnaire. A more holistic psychology asks: 'What is it like to be this other person; to have lived their life? What is the meaning and significance, for them, of this distress? What is the meaning and significance, for them, of me, now? What needs do I need to address that they might not (yet) be able to articulate? Answers are hardly to be found in academically studied or managerially designated psychologies. Only a personally imaginative and engaged sentience can lead us to bespoke compassion.

Isn't all this just overcomplicated and academic? No.

Why, then, is it important? Because our conventionally assumed or conferred language and knowledge largely configure our pattern of understanding and engagement with others. How we think, speak and document will determine what we do. If our language eschews personal resonance and understanding, our actions will follow suit. Any System, in excess, will offer specious clarity and certainty. We must be vigilant; an overreaching scientism will become a pyrrhic progress. Overusing the language, understanding and interventions of disease in the territory of dis-ease is such a seductive but debilitating error. Like a mislocated expedition, it leads to a massive misapplication of effort and resources. Not only does this lose us efficiency and economy. The loss of personal understanding is even more serious: unnecessary attribution of illness mentality and behaviour can be profoundly disempowering. Myopic and inapt labelling generates its own disabilities. The loss of personal language, autonomy, agency and responsibility – these are all causes and casualties of an over-reaching medical model. In our preoccupation to measure we often deskill and desensitise ourselves in the unmeasurable. A mind full of generic dicta, data and algorithms cannot heed the individual voice.

Such losses can largely account for the recurrently exposed, shocking and grotesque examples of basic failures of care in hospitals – institutions which are heavily invested with high-technology and managed care-pathways.

We are faced with a serious and perennial conundrum: in our muscular but blind resolve to treat, we may easily destroy the gentler sentience to heal and humanely care. Compassion may be powerful in effect, but it is fragile in viability: it needs a mindful and respectful space and ambience to survive.

2. Healthcare is important and complicated. All practitioners should be tightly monitored and controlled. Increasing healthcare management is bound to be to the patient's benefit.

Yes, but only sometimes. The caveats for this are broadly similar to the section above. For example, the rules and regulations addressing safety in a Cardiac Surgery Unit should be strictly enforced. Exceptions would be very exceptional, if ever. In contrast, such tight governance is much less helpful when attempting to relieve functional complaints. For example, a perfectionistic lonely person with tension headaches, or another incapacitated by rage and grief at the discovery of a major infidelity, or another enervated by mysterious polysymptoms since his wife became pregnant. In these functional disorders, the therapeutic effect of the practitioner depends upon imaginative skills of personal contact and suggestion. Institutional or formulaic management are likely to run counter to these: rigid management eviscerates compassionate imagination.

There are parallels here to family-life and how we bring up children. The balance we choose between rules *v* freedom and structure *v* spontaneity, etc, will vary with the child, its age, the situation, and so forth. Families where structure and discipline are rigid and excessive will yield children who may appear orderly and well behaved, but are stunted in their capacities for creativity, initiative, expression, joy and intimacy. Necessary conflict, too, will be turned inwards or displaced, with all the destructive effects within and without.

Organisations that are over-managed show equivalent afflictions. Such harassed groups suffer from defensive proceduralism, low-morale, high sickness rates, scapegoating, and a fascinatingly subtle range of subversion, both conscious and unconscious. Paradoxically, such depletions are retroflected casualties; the result of management compulsively 'driving' efficiency. Over-controlling parents rarely get what they intend. Compassion, too, requires our intelligent flexibility.

3. Mass-production and standardization must be a good thing, if it makes things more available.

We don't question this with washing-machines or ball-bearings. Entering the arena of healthcare, we can still extend this confidence to, say, pharmaceuticals, surgical materials and certain procedural treatments, eg cataract extraction. This remains true so long as individual variation, subjective complexity and personal understanding are relatively uninfluential. In contrast, chronic and functional complaints confront us with the importance of individuals' variation of experience and meaning. These all-too-human factors elude quantitative, formulaic and procedural approaches. We must here develop more flexible, 'crafted' and individually addressed responses. Centrally-programmed factory workers are not equipped for this. What are these elusive variables, and how are they important?

Much of this we know from everyday experience. For example, most of us, when distressed by personal or relationship problems, find difficulty in describing, expressing or explaining these. We are likely to have all kinds of fears about sharing or disclosure. How a listener or helper might respond becomes decisive as to whether and how we do this. In this process we are exquisitely sensitive to the subtlest interpersonal signals and changes. Example: how we feel with apparently tiny variations of voice, timing or body language with a verbal greeting or a handshake. For all their power, such nuances of interpersonal influence are almost impossible to measure or manage directly. Paradoxically, though, over-management may stifle, even extinguish, an emotionally-literate environment, which creatively respects the fragile complexity and uniqueness of each interchange. Compassion needs space and oxygen to flourish. Analogies with parenting are, again, clear and prophetic.

4. Competition, commissioning and commercial pressures will raise standards of care.

In industry, encouragement of these '3Cs' makes much sense: in providing technical services and physical commodities, and the manufacture and sale of objects. With complex welfare activities it, again, leads to a similar pattern of the unintended. The '3Cs' solution often becomes more problematic than the problem it is attempting to address. For example, if we attempt to commodify, and then trade, in 'packages of care', how do we pre-scribe the changing, often inexplicit, complexity of people's needs? And then any need for flexibility and sensitivity of response? How do we then standardise a package and a price? If we mandate such specification, what is the human cost of doing so?

To illustrate such problems:

Mr C is 62 years and needs a total hip replacement due to premature osteoarthritis. He is otherwise very fit, healthy, happy and actively involved in his work and large family.

Mrs D is 83 years and also needs this operation. She is a childless widow: she had a stillbirth 60 years ago and never again conceived. Her beloved husband died of cancer a year ago. She now lives alone; lonely, with stoic and brave melancholy. She was an only child and was sexually abused:

she is wary of any kind of physical care or examination. Her complex diabetes and emphysema add to her vulnerability, but she tends to deny this due to her aversion to any kind of dependency.

Clearly, Mrs D's anaesthesia, surgery, physical recovery and psychological resilience are all more likely to be problematic than Mr C's. All these processes will require intelligent and imaginative care. How can such delicate compassion be predictively and commercially contained, controlled or costed? How do we have 'diagnoses' for such kaleidoscopic but decisive human complexity? How will each separate Specialty or Trust precisely delineate and invoice its responsibilities?

What happens with a system of competitive commissioning? Practitioners become controlled by their thraldom to Trusts, and the Trusts are in thrall to optimising their profits and 'performance data'. Thus are they likely to fulfil to the letter (only) their contractual obligations. Officious practice flourishes; managers, even lawyers, direct and tailor individual practice to suit institutional and commercially negotiated 'contracts', and thus policies. These replace more humanistic or holistic practice: encounters guided by broader and longer-term views, and informed by a growing understanding of each particular individual.

Under such a system, over time, we lose vocational practitioners: those motivated primarily by the pursuit of humane enquiry and healing relationships. These become replaced by 'Teams' of management-directed, piece-work biomechanics. Chosen vocations become managed careers. Thinking and activity turn institutional, not interpersonal. Resources become increasingly commandeered for defensive and offensive organisational fights and feints: meetings about meetings – negotiation, litigation, imposing but slyly tendentious statistics, PR, 'spin'... Services that for several decades existed in a state of trusting and cooperative confederation, now become mistrustful competitors: Trusts (!).

The patient is now a commercial proposition: if he generates revenue (for the Trust), then find reasons to provide a service; if he does not generate revenue, then find reasons swiftly to discharge him somewhere (anywhere) else. 'It's not our responsibility.'

Amidst this Darwinian struggle for survival, can our compassion really be commissioned or commodified?

5. Specialisation is always a good thing. It provides greater expertise when and where it is needed

Yet again this is most impressively true with well-defined structural disease, but often counter-productive when dealing with more complex and less stable situations. Positive examples of the use of specialisation are clear and obvious. If we have a knee problem that requires surgery, then we want, not just an orthopaedic surgeon, but one who specialises in knees. The idea is that we can divide the body up into smaller and smaller parts and systems, and thus concentrate knowledge, effort and expertise with greater precision and efficiency. This is viable so long as we are dealing with disease that is stable and confined to a body-part or system. We can term this fragmenting specialisation 'Anatomisation'.

This kind of specialisation can become far from helpful when applied away from the stable, localised disease scenario. To illustrate:

Mr S is age 70 years. Two years ago he developed an aggressive form of Parkinson's Dementia, shortly after his retirement. He had been an extremely educated, fit, diligent and disciplined man, holding a senior post in international diplomacy. His multidimensional decline has been relentless and tragic. He has become an insentient and incontinent shell of his former self, recognising no one and requiring constant care. Amidst this, his beleaguered, self-sacrificing wife discovers a breast-lump, a cancer. She then has chemoradiotherapy, which itself makes her ill, in the hope of a cure. As Mrs S struggles to recover, Mr S's decline is unabated. He has unmanageable 'episodes': he freezes, falls, develops chest infections, deepening deliria. Each of these needs his admission to hospital, and each time it is to a different Ward and a different 'Team', who do not recognise him. Each team then routinely refers him on to further specialist teams: to Gerontology (for his age!), to Neurology (for Parkinson's), to Elderly Psychiatry (for Dementia), to Urology (for recurrent urine infections), to Respiratory Medicine (for chest infections). None of these teams seems to acknowledge the larger picture, and what is needed in terms of wise, humane contact; continuity, containment support and comfort. Mrs S is an intelligent woman, but now fatigued, despondent and confused by the constantly changing medical personnel, designations and venues.

'Why does he need yet another brain scan?', she wearily asks a bustling and brisk Neurology Registrar.

'Just to make sure we're not missing anything', comes his clipped reply, his tone of defensive authority primed by Trust Protocol.

Thirty years ago this unneeded and very expensive brain scan would not have been available. Nor would the panoply of specialist teams. Mr and Mrs S would have had something else: continuity of care by a known general physician on a particular ward. This broadly-based clinician and dedicated nursing staff would have provided the personal investment, familiarity, acknowledgement and understanding that were needed to nurse and palliate all of these 'episodes'. They would have seamlessly apprehended the human needs, not just of the ravaged Mr S, but also his exhausted wife. They would probably not have used the word 'compassion', but it would have been woven into their experiences, acts and utterances. Such traditional skills are easily displaced by the often specious imperative to 'specialisation'. The whole is more than the sum of its parts: compassion is a tender and fragile fruit of holism.

Ms T is a 38-year-old single woman with a son of four years. Her persona of engaging warmth and polite cooperation belies her deeply troubled and troubling history. A product and victim of, and hostage to, a painfully unhappy parental marriage, she has spent most of her life trying impotently to break free, to establish an autonomous and wholesome self. But she has not the self-esteem, the internal model, or sense of entitlement to do any of these things. She is like a blinded, enraged, captive creature convulsively throwing itself against the bars of its cage, trying to find the outside. The symptoms signalling this impacted struggle have been wide-ranging. They have been shepherded and clustered by a parade of specialists over many years: mood disturbance and instability, gastritis, eating disorders, intermittent alcoholism, impulsivity, irritable bowel syndrome, obsessive compulsive disorder, migraines, menstrual dysfunction, eczema...

Each specialist attempted to subsume, quell, or at least contain, her disturbance with their own language and circumscribed focus of the medical model. Sometimes, paradoxically, such specialisation led to her being the object of exclusion instead: once she was lost between the GP Counsellor, the Psychiatric and the Alcohol Services, who each said that one of the others should be responsible. Despite seeking helpful engagement, she was extruded by all three: 'she does not meet our intake criteria'; 'It's not our responsibility...'

Dr W, her General Practitioner, has learned over many years that such marathon, polymorphous disturbance is usually signalling some failure of personal evolution, some frustration of gratified belonging. It lies behind and beyond any specialisms, their language or measurements. He remembers an old mentor saying of his endeavours to help such people: 'You need patience with patients, and patients with patience'. But Dr

W knows now that it requires also evocative but structured encouragement, to safely uncover and decipher what lies beneath. He arranges an hour's appointment with Ms T, to try to take them both from a world of fragmented and serial specialisms, to a holistic perspective deriving from, and imbued with, personal meaning.

The polyclinic Practice Manager is alerted, and now uneasy: 'We have pressure on clinic rooms, doctor, and this kind of work takes up a lot of time, and earns no additional "points" for the Practice ... in any case, all the other doctors have said this kind of work is not your responsibility ...'

*

Is there a more crystalline coda for these Five Follies?

*

And the question arising? In a healthcare system increasingly determined by the quantifiable, the commercial and the industrial, how do we restore, and then assure, the primacy of holistic, human care – the quality and continuity of our personal contact with others? In our busy and difficult jobs, every day and in every consultation, how do we create afresh, then nurture, an ever-evanescent culture of compassion?

*

'Is it progress if a cannibal eats with a knife and fork?'

Stanislaw Lec, *Unkempt Thoughts*, 1962

*

APPENDIX

	Disease	Dis-ease
1. Knowledge	Impersonal Objective, generic, clustered, data	Personal Subjective/ intersubjective, Idiomorphic, bespoke
2. Ideology/ paradigm	Dualism, Determinism, Biomechanics	Monism, choice, consciousness
3. Resources/ transmission	External (eg drugs, instruments, radiation, manipulation, lasers) By Conduction 'Treatment'	Internal (eg immunity, growth, repair) By Induction 'Healing'
4.Power/ responsibility	Dr >>> Pt	Pt [+/-Dr]
5. Language	Objective, Doctors', technical, designatory Generic	(Inter)personal. Shared dialogue = co-creation Idiolectic
6.Communication mode	Didactic Mostly logical/structured	Dialogue/Dialectic Often openly imaginative/ evocative
7. Psychology	Designatory 'Objective' Quantitatively researched	Evocative (Inter)subjective Qualitatively researched
8. Role/ metaphor of Doctor/healer	Engineer, expert, teacher, manager	Gardener, guide, midwife, compassionate fellow-traveller

9. Art or Science?	Science	Art
10. Accessibility to industrialisation: mass-management, , training, standardisation, mass production, commodification, measurement	High	Low
11. Importance of personal contact, meaning and understanding	Low	High

Figure 1: Disease v. Dis-ease; Art and Science, Treatment and Healing: comparative paradigms of effective response to human ailments

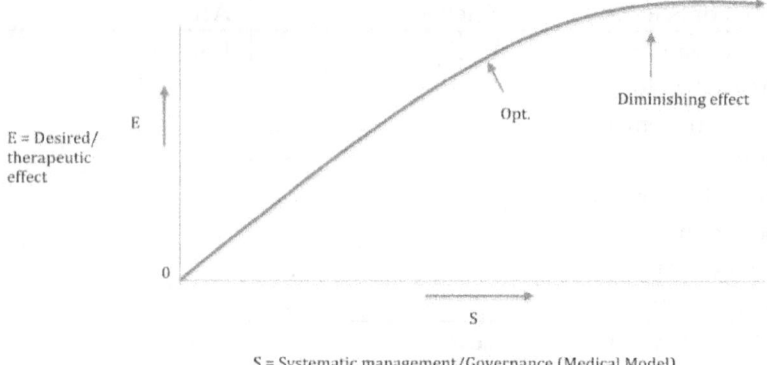

S = Systematic management/Governance (Medical Model)

Figure 2: Systematic management and structural disease
Decaying exponential. Desired response proportional to systematic governance, until optimal point (Opt). Then diminishing returns. (Illustrated principle: structural disease responds relatively well to scientific strictures and structures.)

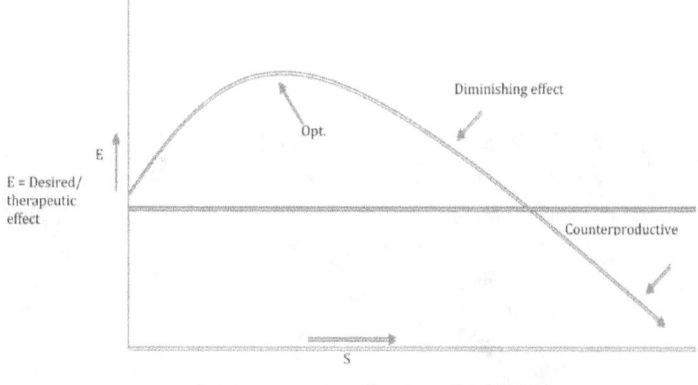

Figure 3: Systematic/generic management and functional dis-ease Shallower Bell Curve with reversal. Desired response to systematic governance is less. Yields earlier to ineffectiveness, then becomes counterproductive. (Illustrated principle: functional dis-ease less positively responsive to impersonally prescribed approaches. Excess application has adverse effects.)

Ω

Submitted to the Secretary of State for Health. It was subsequently published in the *Journal of Holistic Healthcare*, Vol 8. Issue 3. Dec 2011.

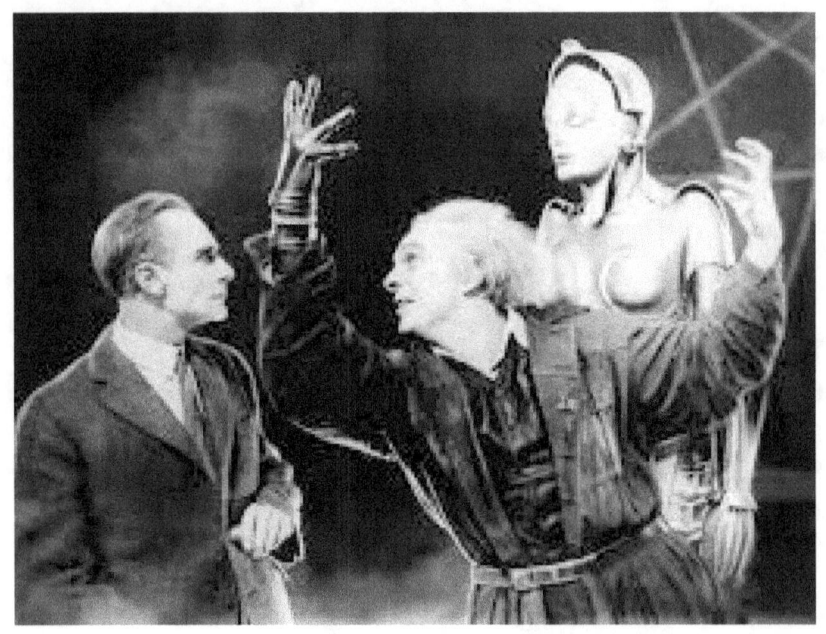

Fritz Lang *Metropolis 1927*

Further NHS Reforms: inevitable and unintended Consequences

As the debate becomes more fraught, I want to add my voice to the fray. I have been a frontline Medical Practitioner for more than forty years, and have seen recurrent waves of reform and their very mixed results. The least disputable advances are in the realms of technology and technical competence: drugs and procedures have become more accurate and effective, practitioners mostly apposite in their delivery. Likewise, a few decades ago we all knew of doctors widely reputed as rude, curt, alcoholic, incompetent and shabby – sometimes simultaneously. In those times, with moderate luck, they would retire, without formal challenge, on a full NHS Pension. That kind of collusive incompetence is now most unlikely. These changes represent real progress.

But the institutional reconfigurations and the management devices applied to achieve these have inadvertently destroyed much of the best, in order to extirpate the worst. I experienced this 'best' in my first twenty-five years, working in NHS General Practice and Psychiatry. I was mentored by Practitioners who were vocational in their ethos and holistic in their view of their specialty. Although my administrative duties and salary were referable to one tiny sector of the NHS, my professional efforts and communications roamed with easy and pragmatic conviviality amongst colleagues from other disciplines and institutions. Despite some 'bad' practitioners, I felt mostly a welcoming and fraternal support: a kind of 'therapeutic family'. I was not then much interested in branded politics, but I wondered if this was one of the few good and viable examples of a kind of 'Confederate Socialism': a world of colleagial exchanges that was benignly intentioned, inclusively respectful and often mutually educational and supportive.

'Medicine is a humanity guided by science': not a phrase I heard explicitly from my early mentors, but they would have readily agreed.

For the last two decades this network of interpersonal communication, support and understanding has been increasingly eroded and dismantled by various ideas to increase 'efficiency'. The galvanising panoply has included: The Internal Market; Commissioning; NHS Trusts; the widening of schematic medicalisation of complex human distress; mandating goals and targets, performance-related pay and league tables; proliferation of ever more and sharply defined specialties, then acceleration of specialist training … and now GP Commissioning. The danger with each and all of these is that Medical Practice is propelled away from any basis as a humanely networked welfare activity, and towards an entrepreneurial kind of 'civic engineering' whose currency is commodification. Thus, increasingly, we attempt to 'manage' people and their distress without the commensurate growth of personal contact, meaning and understanding.

Notions and methods from commerce and manufacturing industries may make some useful contributions to Healthcare, but they are seriously limited. Beyond these limits they can do real damage. NHS doctors' pay and working hours are now more generous than twenty years ago; in contrast, their morale, work-satisfaction and sense of creative and compassionate engagement (with colleagues, as well as patients) are not. In a recent large meeting of senior colleagues, we were being briefed and instructed, yet again, by another executive imperative, about a complex and subtle area of care. I protested, saying I felt like an eight-year-old working in a car factory. The identification was explosive and rapturous – especially, I thought, from older colleagues schooled in the earlier culture. The comic relief was evident and welcome. The underlying reservoir of alienation, resentment, mistrust, fear and anomie remains largely unarticulated, and little understood.

Doctors are probably the most privileged among the victims of our misindustrialisation of healthcare: certainly they are the best paid. Among other welfare and NHS Healthcare workers the pay is less, but the psycho-spiritual affliction much the same. The shocking stories of elderly, frail, dry-mouthed patients lying with abject helplessness in soiled sheets, while within yards of them nurses sit rapt in electronic engagement with abstracted NHS Foundation Trust data collation tasks, are harsh symptoms of a malign Zeitgeist: the consequences of depersonalising the personal. This is what happens when we overinvest in the biomechanical, when we industrialise the procedural, but fail to see or value or understand the complexity of human needs and attachments.

The biomechanical is necessary but not sufficient in healthcare. Competition, commercialisation and commodification – the 3Cs – may contribute peripherally and in minor ways. But we must heal as well as treat; compassionately engage as well as manage. For these we need practitioners and networks fuelled and nourished by the energy and art of the interpersonal: by humanism and holism. For all its flaws (many otherwise remediable), the old NHS of 'Confederate Socialism' encouraged this in me and for me, and those around me, for twenty-five years.

I am asked: what would I now do to rehumanise our healthcare? To start, I suggest a phased, radical retreat, then reclamation. Practical examples: to abolish any kind of Internal Market, Commissioning, and thus the likes of NHS Foundation Trusts; to restore Hospital Nursing Schools, the centrality of General Physicians, and personal patient lists to General Practitioners. But the cultural tides propelling our problematic recent changes are wide and strong: the easiest course is confluence, to be swept along. Creative counterculture will always be harder.

Amidst these conundra, as my own career nears its end, I mourn the loss of Love's Labour. I fear, too, for my future: when I become old and helpless, what kind of personal care and understanding will I receive?

Ω

Letter to the *British Medical Journal* 2012

'Evidence' is both more and less than it seems

The rise of scientism and the demise of the personal in healthcare

Dear Mr Hunt MP

(Secretary of State for Health 2012)

I am writing to you as a long-serving single-handed GP: now an almost-extinct species, but one occupying an exceptional vantage point for length and familiarity. My views, therefore, often have a different emphasis from many of the consulted professional bodies.

I heard a recent interview with you (Radio 4, 19/10/12) in which you talked of 'being led by scientific evidence'. The phrase can sound unarguably sensible and pragmatic: in healthcare it has become increasingly used as a kind of justifying slogan or even shibboleth: measure or perish. But the words 'evidence' and 'led' may be trickier than we realise: a brief analysis may clarify.

Evidence is a highly complex endeavour; its complexity grows with scrutiny. Some general principles can help us navigate: evidence occupies a spectrum of contentiousness – it is much clearer with the inanimate than the human. And with the human it is much clearer with the objectively physical than the experiential. To help tether all this we have quantifiable evidence, and this is often regarded as a 'gold-standard' of clarity and certainty. Yet in complex human healthcare it is often difficult (sometimes impossible) to quantify what we are really interested in without introducing speciousness of many kinds. Nevertheless quantifiable evidence now commands such high cultural-currency value that much 'counterfeit-currency' is produced and sought; this 'bad currency' then enters our exchanges to displace an intelligent openness to other kinds of (unquantifiable) evidence.

What does this lead to?

In my view the most serious adverse changes are those of the loss of personal attachments and their understandings. Because these are mostly impossible to measure, standardise or regulate, they cannot be readily turned into the staples of current NHS managed operations: statistical data, standardised procedures or tradable commodities. Efforts to do so are now frequent and have often grotesquely absurd consequences: difficult and detailed questionnaires given to the rawly distressed from life-shock or bereavement; poorly understood children from painfully struggling families being didactically diagnosed with 'neurodevelopmental disorders' – these are common follies from our growing medical scientism.

In earlier times – before the ubiquity of computers and our consequent submission to the quantified and the mass-managed – it was far easier for health carers to develop attachments and personal understandings. These were often of great therapeutic value. Good practice then recognised that our capacity to heal, contain or comfort depend on professionally tempered attachments and affections: the better we know people, the better we can care for them. Current trends obstruct such possibilities: rapid rotations of staff and venues, multiple 'hit and run' specialists, generic and anonymised teams rather than named and familiar persons ... With complex and chronic ailments, in particular, these 'management systems' cannot readily offer compassionate and imaginative containment.

The culture of healthcare has rapidly and radically changed. We have incrementally displaced the ethos of a family with that of a factory: personal connections and understandings are increasingly rare; standardised procedures and utterances common. Far fewer people know the name of their GP; in their large Polyclinics GPs cannot personally remember their patients and do not even know the names of their own receptionists. In the large district hospitals Consultants do their ward-rounds with junior medical staff they have never met before, often, seeing patients for a first and only time. Patients – often alone, exposed and afraid – feel unable to express their vulnerability and needs to rule-bound and management-programmed nurses. Such anomie has burgeoned in parallel with the regal rise, then hegemony, of (quantifiable) evidence. This is not coincidental. Yet we also know that our best relationships are largely fuelled by certain kinds of faith, aspiration and ideal – and that none of these could be quantitatively 'evidenced'. We live with gratitude and wonder for such indeterminate anomalies: our faith lies at the heart of our humanity.

This brings me back to your use of the word 'led': for we should rarely be led by scientific evidence, rather we should be guided. This means we guard and retain our autonomy so that we may be informed by much else, too. For we need our broadest understandings; we need to be able to discern, and yet assimilate, very different kinds of comprehension and knowledge. In healthcare, as in much of life, wisdom is often the conciliation and choreography of options that are themselves inescapably flawed or limited.

My own slogan is 'Healthcare is a humanity guided by science'. The implication here reminds us to be, always, careful and mindful of such delicate balances and conundra. This is not easy, yet to avoid such complexity leads to what we have now: a healthcare rich in provided resources, but cumulatively impoverished of internally generated human connection and understanding.

My voice is experienced, though old: I hope you find some freshness in the views. It would interest me greatly to continue a dialogue. If you, or one of your deputies, want to visit my inner London GP practice you can see In Vivo what has motivated and informed this letter.

Ω

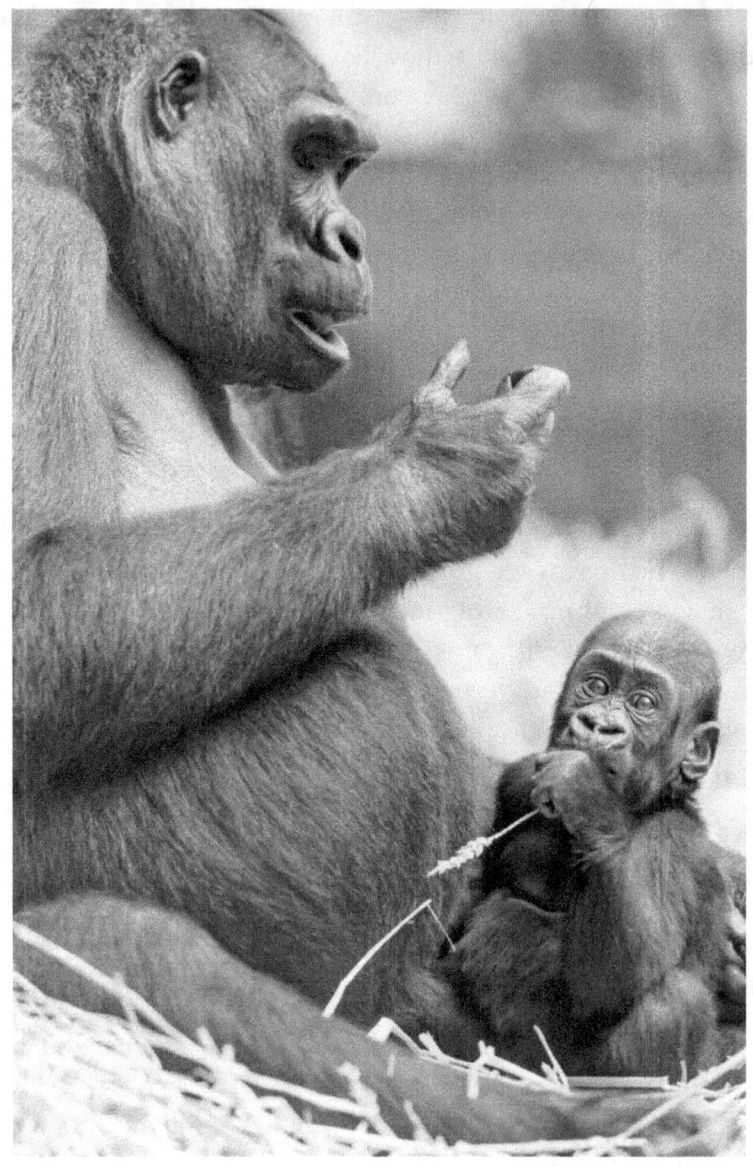

Continuity of Care -
Of course, but whose?

A Sleight of Slogans
– letter to Family Doctor Association

Continuity of Care is a phrase increasingly used to indicate a cornerstone of good practice. But the phrase is often used with very different assumptions and intent: personal and institutional continuity are often discordant. Personal care and family-doctoring are both an art and an ethos: we must beware of ultimately expensive and mass-produced imitations.

Names and titles quickly convey a designation, sometimes evaluation. Similarly, slogans attempt to transmit a message – often moral or transformative – with sharp economy, sometimes wit. Sloganeers aim to rapidly catch our interest and affiliation.

And so it was. Some years ago I was 'caught' by the title of The Small Practices Association (SPA): I joined. I was – and resolutely remain – a well-defined, small practice. Single-handed in London's centre, I sensed the rising cultural tides running against me. I steeled myself: I would have to be articulate and resilient to guard and nourish the kind of personal understandings and relationships that have been at the heart of my working lifetime's vocation. Long experience has fuelled my conviction that a small practice is best suited to the delivery of person-centred healthcare. The SPA's title vaunted (and provided) valuable support to stand against the tide.

In more recent years the SPA rebranded itself as the Family Doctor Association, the current FDA. I liked this title, too. For my work is much enriched when I can see and understand an individual's struggles and afflictions within broader frames of life-cycles and relationships: a family-perspective is essential to this. There are here some interesting and daunting parallels. In earlier years I experienced my work as being part of the broader endeavours of a kind of colleagial healthcare 'family' – in this some individuals were close and well-known, others invisible and unknown – an extended 'family', nevertheless. Sadly, for expedient organisational then cultural reasons, doctors now usually have much less personal knowledge of patients and families, and are less likely in their work to feel affiliated into a national healthcare 'family' Both kinds of family-contact in our work are impoverished.

I mourn the loss of these subtle personal nexi. I see and fear the consequences. But there is restitution – the FDA's slogan, Continuity of Care, enlivens and encourages me: it draws from timeless principles of healing. These principles help us revise and revitalise a healthcare that is increasingly anonymised, alienated, algorithmetised – a culture that has steadily lost any individual view of people in its exponential development of the schematic and managerial. For any real reconciliation here, we need to exert a kind of healing. Central to healing processes are two triads. One develops within the individual (the intrapersonal): immunity, growth and repair. This first triad is induced by a second, which develops between individuals (the interpersonal): attachment, containment and affection.

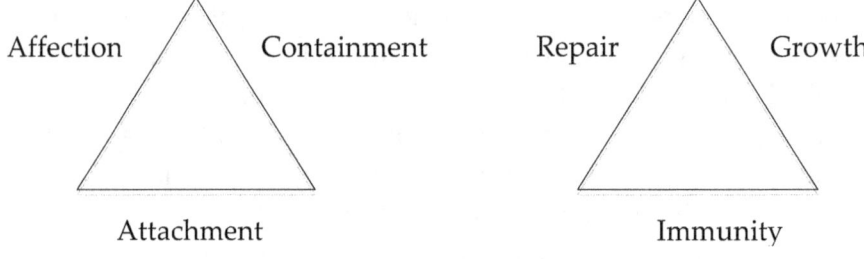

Affection   Containment   Repair   Growth

Attachment   Immunity

Figure 1:	**Figure 2:**
Interpersonal healing inductions	*Intrapersonal healing inductions*
The 'family' *ethos* of	The 'family' *effects* of
well-fared welfare	well-fared welfare
Difficult to measure	Difficult to measure
Personal	Personal

Clearly, for any of these to occur, the presence of good therapeutic rapport is likely to be crucial. How can these things evolve without continuity of care? This seems a rhetorical question.

The professional responses, though, are less straightforward; we need to look carefully.

'Continuity of Care' can be constructed very differently by, say, patients, administrators and different sorts of doctors. Personal continuity is the familiar face, voice and ambience: the uniquely evolved complex of contacts, events and personal understandings. This kind of continuity is what we yearn for when a condition renders us vulnerable because of its chronicity and complexity. If we live long enough we all suffer this vulnerability, and will seek succour in personal familiarity and continuity. This succour often has a kind of organic growth, for the nourishing and warming benefits to patients of personal continuity are often equally important to practitioners. For the more humanly interested doctor, it is the relationships that keep heart and mind alive, fresh, engaged and integrated. And here is a powerful and wonderful mystery: caring for those that matter to us adds to our own lives and energies.

But there is a very different ethos of continuity of care that is increasingly vaunted by planners, managers and, now, a new generation of practitioners. This emphasises institutional and administrative impersonal continuity: here it is the designated 'Team' that delivers; any desire for personal attachment is discouraged. Personal understanding becomes an obsolescent and irrelevant impediment: data is the official currency. The intention is that anonymised healthcare professionals and patients can all be speedily referred to managed Services Care Pathways and Team Protocols. These administrative devices attempt to template a kind of in loco parentis for personally responsible and responsive care. This will, of course, take us far away from care anchored in the personally familiar. Where, then, does all this lead? Here are two examples:

Suki has deep-rooted dysthymic mental health problems that cannot be simply 'treated', even less 'cured'. Her early childhood was rent and wounded by unstable, inconsistent and incompetent parenting. What seems to work for her – very slowly – is the reverse of all these in her healthcare: kindness, consistency, patience, imaginative and respectful interest. As her GP I try to provide this by offering my personal continuity of care: her appreciation of this is subtly evident and demurely expressed.

Nevertheless, she gets mentally ill, and this is when attachments fragment and unravel. In one turbulent year she encountered the following psychiatric teams: Hospital Liaison Psychiatry, Community Mental Health, Assertive Outreach, Emergency Psychiatry, Crisis Resolution, Home Treatment, In-Patient Psychiatry, Early Discharge and Recovery. Each of these boundaried teams transferred electronic abstracted 'data' to the next team, to prime their very long and formulaic assessment. The electronic continuity might seem seamless and neatly well-functioning to a manager or detached clinician. Suki's experience is shockingly and instructively different. At the times when she most needs familiar and trusted faces, and attachments rooted in personal knowledge, she instead encounters a procession of strangers who interrogate her, often never to be seen again. She describes these often stilted disquisitions as if they are conducted for an unseen third person, but not really for her. She rarely remembers their names or designations.

I tell some senior managers and clinicians what I have heard and seen. They diplomatically imply that my view is lacking in clarity and sophistication. They tell me that Suki is the recipient of a well-honed system of 'Integrated Care': she is being managed through her 'Patient Journey'; the procession of strangers are, in fact, choreographed specialists, each tending a complex niche in this engineered journey. I think: whose language and needs are being heeded? And who decides?

I have had a part-time hospital post for many years. Much of my work has been to help patients with complex interweavings of substantial physical disease and emotional distress. I have heard patients' accounts of their medical encounters for decades. Until recent times, patients would almost always know who their GP was: often the rapport was deep, trusted and clearly valued. This is now very rare: most frequently patients know the names of their health centre, but not any particular doctor. 'I used to see Dr J, but now when I go it always seems to be someone different ... the last time it was a young woman: she seemed nice enough but spent most of the time looking on the screen. No, I don't know her name ...' This is typical of our increasing healthcare data-centred anonymity.

This serious loss of personal attachment has been accelerated by the abolition of Personal Patient Lists. This administrative fiat discouraged the development of particular personal bonds and replaces them with Systemic Management; when I now go to my GP I am not to think of myself as cared for by my doctor, Dr X: my care is now managed by the Hillside Primary Care Medical Centre.

There are essential differences between these contrapuntal kinds of continuity of care: the personal and the administrative. Generally planners and managers will favour and better understand administrative and systemic continuity as this can be (theoretically) delivered with detachment and objectivity. Clearly, these kinds of continuity must always be available – for no individual practitioner can provide invariable, eternal, perfect and instant personal care, or not for long! We must all be allowed absences, holidays, and the errors and vicissitudes of life. Yes, personal continuity can rarely be complete and there must always be institutional back-up plans and resources.

So, we must have both kinds of continuity of care: personal and impersonal. The problem then is how do we define, find and assure the best mix or compromise in each situation? Certain principles can guide us. Where a patient and practitioner wish for personal continuity of care for a non-acute condition – and this possibility is feasible and competent – then this should take precedence. Yet this personal continuity should be contained within, and in some ways accountable to, a systemic continuity: this is the safety-net, lest the personal continuity breaks or fails.

None of this is easy. In our risk-averse times we have become haunted by spectres of breakage and failure. And personal continuity of care – like love – is vulnerable to loss and damage. Yet to attempt to avoid these risks – by driving out personal attachments and replacing them with 'safer' generic management – may lead to different, but greater, breakages and failures. Broken spirits and hearts are common and often ineluctably important in our health and welfare. Such complex humanity eludes management and measurement: at these times we need a harbour of experienced compassion and imagination. Skilled and personal continuity of care may be the best kind of harbour we can offer.

It is better to have loved and lost,
than never to have loved at all.

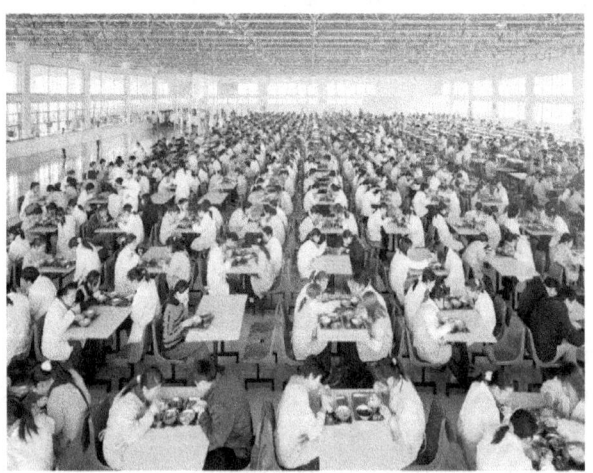

Ω

Publ. in *Family Doctor 2012*

Balancing Healthcare
Technical v. Personal
Local v. Systemic

Closures at Lewisham Hospital

I heard your important but brief debate on BBC Radio 4 on 26 January. As expected, your arguments were cogent, though polarised. What was not explicated was the inescapable conundra we now have in contemporary healthcare: that there are, increasingly, juxtaposed principles we must balance – these are technical vs personal, objective vs (inter)subjective and science vs art. The conundra arise most clearly when we cannot easily combine these, when they remain antithetical: then we need the wisdom of our best compromises. As you have demonstrated, finding the right balance is no easy task.

I am a long-serving, small-practice City GP with an attentive view of people and their relationships. I think we have a growing problem – paradoxically – from the indisputable success of the scientific/technical/objective in certain areas: because of these successes they have largely hegemonised our mindsets, budgets and plans in all areas of healthcare. This has then led to an inadvertent neglect of the personal/art/(inter)subjective in healthcare: people! We have lost our balance and this is now manifest in our healthcare centres being often technology-rich but humanity-poor: shock headlines pillory the worst examples, but it is clear to me that this sinister new pattern has much to teach us.

Yes, of course it is important that we receive the best technical care, but we must attempt to do so in a humanly-scaled and responsive milieu, where people feel seen, heard, understood, connected and cared-for. These interactions are complex living processes which can only survive with the interpersonal equivalents of space, oxygen, nutrients and habitat. For these we need a 'family' environment, if we are to perform our 'factory' tasks with rooted and growing humanity.

Yes, larger regionalised Specialist Units may logistically provide better technical care, but how do we combine high volumes of technically exacting and urgently required work (that is needed for the procedures of treatment) with a personal sense of connection and understanding (that is required for the care of healing)? For when we industrialise healthcare to treat more efficiently, the care often drains away. If we are not mindful of this, it becomes inevitable.

If we take the examples of Stroke, or Coronary Care, it may make good sense to centralise and specialise skills and expensive resources, and this is probably reflected in good results. But results will be better still if personal connections and communications are regarded as an equal priority. This is even more so with chronic conditions. The required balance of centralised efficiency vs locality identifications needs careful thought: it may be very different for different people.

This is now a formidable task as the personally connected aspects of the NHS have suffered from inadvertent but parlous selective inattention. I now work in a health service where, increasingly, patients cannot name their GP or hospital consultant, doctors have little personal knowledge or understanding of their patients, colleagues do not know one another, Hospital Consultants do ward rounds with junior staff and nurses they do not know, seeing patients for a first and only time ... There are many more examples. What kind of therapeutic contacts, affections or care can develop in such a system? What happens to staff morale? Our shock-headlines provide a darker part of the answer.

The causes of such industrialised healthcare casualties are numerous, complex and sometimes obscure. The fact that very large organisations with rapid human throughput may have difficulty in positively bonding with and understanding complexly distressed individuals may be easy to discern and explain. Other decisions and events which alienate, depersonalise, dislocate and demoralise may be more obscure, but just as real. Examples? The dispersal of hospital nursing schools to Universities; the European Working Hours Directive; the amalgamation of smaller, identity-rich Medical Schools; the abolition of GP personal lists; the economic discouragement of small GP practices; the demise of the General Physician – all such have contributed to our ever more tightly managed, but anomic, healthcare.

How we reinfuse and re-enthuse our often misindustrialised healthcare with human heart and professional art, is an endless and difficult challenge, for the problems now have deep cultural roots. If we can discern our excessive uses of industrialisation, informatics, systems management, competition, commodification and commercialisation, we may be able to act with more intelligent restraint. Those smaller, more fragile and imperilled, caring aspects of healthcare may then revive and, possibly, flourish.

Small and large, generic and bespoke, art and science, universal and vernacular, all address different aspects of our complex health needs. We need matching, complex, though pragmatic, responses. There are rarely (if ever) solutions, only our wisest compromises.

I have a distilled slogan for all of this: 'Healthcare is a humanity guided by science'.

Ω

Letter to Joan Ruddock, MP and Lord Ara Darzi (ex Minister of Health) 2013

'Fixing the NHS is straightforward'

Really?

Gerry Robinson in his article (Daily Telegraph, 18.2.13) tells us that 'fixing the NHS is straightforward'. He writes with optimistic alacrity of pragmatic, logistical, data-fuelled managerial devices to sharpen purview and performance. He cites management in McDonalds and Phones4U as good role models for healthcare. He conveys this as if it is bold and new.

I have been a frontline NHS doctor for more than forty years and my view is very different. For in the last two decades we have had ever-increasing infusions of such Management Modelling and Corporate redesigns, based on what works in Commerce and manufacturing industries. The resulting industrialisation of healthcare – and its guidance by the 3Cs: commissioning, competition and commodification – has led to grievous loss of humane interest, attachments and vocation in healthcare. The Mid Staffs debacle is one severe and grotesque consequent example.

My own view has become countercultural. It is that healthcare is a humanity guided by science. That humanity is an art and an ethos; these cannot simply be managed or manufactured. They are complex manifestations of education and culture more than any training and obedience. At the heart of this humanity lie the questions of why and how we should care for one another. The best answers come from milieux that can respectfully grow personal attachments, affections and understandings. The less industrial, older NHS fostered such important subtleties much more readily.

Healthcare is bedevilled by such chimera and complexity. It is dangerous folly to think we can easily short-circuit these by some kind of brilliant, quasi-commercial or military-type plans or charismatic leadership. 'Straightforward'? No. 'Fixes'? There are none: we can offer only our wisest and most compassionate and dextrous compromises. Mid Staffs is not so much about simple managerial incompetence; it is more about the overgrowth of managerialism and the inadvertent asphyxiation of natural humanity.

The older NHS that mentored me may have been less scientifically efficient and managed, but it was richer in humanity and caring imagination.

Ω

Published in BMJ, 2013

The Rise of Business Culture in the NHS:

our consequent loss of compassionate healthcare ethos

I write in agreement with Professor Elkeles' thoughts about the dehumanised disarray in our NHS.

I, too, am a veteran NHS doctor. Thoughtful practitioners of my generation are almost always in agreement: the twenty years' development of the 'internal (healthcare) market' has not enlivened, incentivised or optimised procedural treatments, even less compassionate care. With few exceptions it has led, rather, to widespread staff anomie and demoralisation. As both cause and effect to these we have more depersonalised and formulaic care, managed increasingly in ways that are remote, defensive and officious. The business-modelled NHS costs much more, too: a complexly competitive commissioning system of autarkic Trusts etc leads to an explosion of administrative artefacts and artifices. Healthcare is a humanity: science makes great contributions. But a business? We are discovering just how specious and dangerous this misconception can be. How and why we should care for one another far exceeds any business we can manage.

Ω

Letter to *The Times* 2013

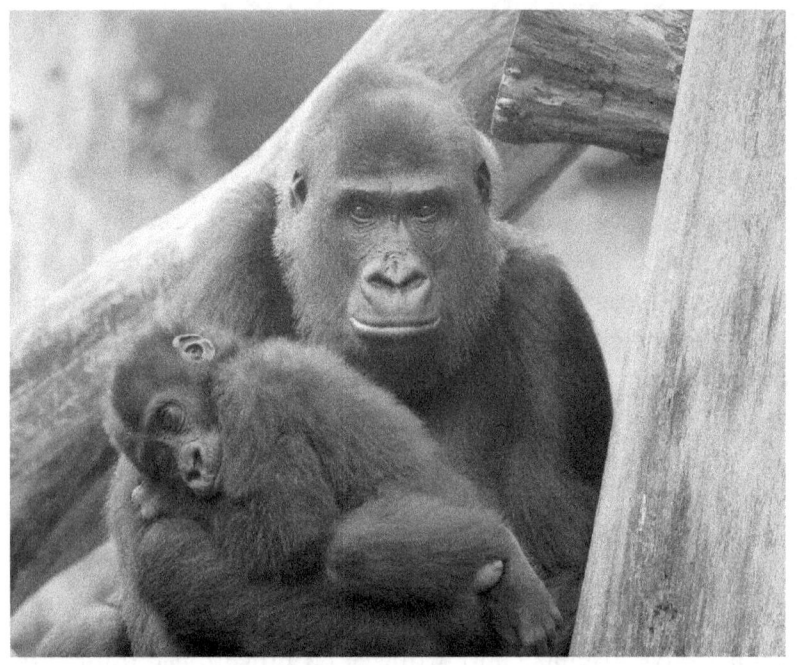

Physis
Healing, Growth and
the Hub of
Personal Continuity of Care

A thirty-nine (39) year delayed
follow-up correspondence with Sally

1. Explanatory introduction

Occasionally benign coincidence far exceeds mere serendipity, as if the cosmos has somehow read and responded to our intent. Receiving the letter was one of those occasions: its primally evocative and illustrative power far exceeds its apparent brevity and plain speaking. This needs some explanation.

First the stage.

For several years I have been increasingly resolute in pursuing qualitative research into the nature and significance of personal continuity of healthcare. I have been led to this by witnessing and enduring the consequences of its progressive loss, especially in the latter third of my professional lifetime. From this has come some understanding. For example, much of this involution derives from the fact that relationships are more difficult to code, manufacture, manage, quantify and research than, say, drugs or physical procedures. This is a conundrum. Rather than acknowledging its difficulty we have instead worsened it by creating something of an academic (then economic and administrative) oligarchy from the 'safer' confines of more easily codifiable and quantifiable research and knowledge – the shibboleths of 'Evidence Basis', a kind of nouveau riche 'Ruling Class'. This newer and narrower culture then often wreaks blind damage because subtle, and thus less measurable, aspects of care then become liable to indifferent neglect or, worse, rationalised hostility and exclusion. In this arena of collateral damage the loss of personal continuity of care is one of the most important and egregious examples. When I was a young practitioner I was encouraged to develop and nurture this earlier longer-term and personal approach. I did not then perceive the probability of its extinction.

Now, the events.

I am perusing a letter, one of many: there are always more. My eyes scan for the sender, semi-consciously, to decide on priority and degree of attention. The name galvanises my distant memory. I then search for other details, to confirm my guess: it is correct.

I have not heard from Sally for thirty-nine years. My visual memory quickly yields her face, its expressions, thence to her mien and spirit; I remember a very sensitive, melancholic and intelligent young woman struggling with her own shadows, intensity and complexity. I cannot remember anything more precise about her symptom-constellation, or her life or family history. I suppose she would be called 'Chronic severe depressive dysthymia': a more adventurous psychiatrist might also risk 'underlying conflicts and struggles with identity formation'.

As I write this I have not refreshed, checked or garnered more details: the account is thus fresh but unrefined. My recollection is that my encounters with Sally spanned about three years and were located in three consecutive Greater London hospitals. I was then a young trainee psychiatrist, very interested in unproceduralised influences of healing. I was certainly receptive to psychotherapeutic ideas but had not (yet) any training. I was only marginally older than Sally and not that differently endowed with resources and problems. I knew this but was able – with care – to sequestrate 'it' but not myself: our roles were then clearly different – our selves and existential predicaments were not. Her letter, after four decades, indicates a further convergence of our common humanity.

Sally's letter is a pithy personal testament of great power and – I believe – importance to all healthcare professionals. Her clear and candid account is suffused with many themes, all of which merit long thought and discussion. I certainly will not attempt to designate these all for the reader, but instead here briefly highlight themes from the cultures of care that include yet transcend we two individuals.

For me, most remarkable is the evidence of how, in those previous decades, we were able to create imaginative, sensitive, flexible services. The best of these could, and did, then deliver a much more substantial person-centred continuity of care. For several years I worked with such services: they are now very rare. I remember my supervisory consultants being accommodating and encouraging to provide the flexibility of arrangements, space and time for this therapeutic relationship (and others) to run its course and bear its fruit. This was possible because there were, then, far fewer diktats, rules and bureaucratic obelisks stymying autonomous, responsible judgements of wisdom and experience. In those days coded and hegemonic psychiatric diagnosis was far less important than personal connection and understanding; care often proceeded down unmade tracks rather than prescribed tarmacked, generic Care Pathways; care was often a delicate dance improvised between individuals rather than an institutional march decreed by academic or administrative committees.

Sally today would be most unlikely to find such continuity of personal containment and accompaniment in any NHS Psychiatric (not Psychotherapy, remember) Services. What she then received may now seem extraordinary, but it was not uncommon then. I am saddened not just for patients, but also for the working welfare of current doctors: few, if any, will have the licence or latitude for such broad, deep or long contact with individuals, or garner the humanly profound and lasting satisfactions.

Some will say that we cannot now economically afford such bespoke services. I do not agree: such care is much cheaper than the kind of anomic, multi-disciplined, multi-teamed approaches that flounder with great expense and poor personal connection in the current NHS. I see this regularly and spend much of my professional time trying to repair the damage. If we do not make good human sense to one another, economic and human costs are much higher.

Sally's letter was a kind of dramatic oxymoron – a shock from the anciently familiar: amidst my current healthcare concerns it rapidly crystallised into a welcome and edifying sense. For the outside reader its private significance for us both is easily imagined. This will produce many individual resonances. Many may identify Agape: non-erotic, unpossessive, unidealised love that is probably essential to Physis. The institutional and cultural themes invite opportunities for reflection that should not be missed: hence this invitation to greater readership. After contact and discussion with Sally she agrees. This is thus a documentary presentation, and to anchor authenticity real names are used.

I have attached my reply to her largely for human interest.

The correspondence is unedited, apart from the omission of addresses. Claybury refers to Claybury Hospital, then a large psychiatric hospital in suburban East London. It closed about twenty years ago.

2. Letter 1

3 June 2013

Dear David Zigmond

Back in the 1970s I was a patient of yours. At first an outpatient at North Middlesex Hospital and then I became an inpatient in Claybury.

I met John at Claybury and although at the time many people advised against us getting together, we went on to have a happy 30 years. Like everyone we had our ups and downs, had three great kids, Rachel, Paul and Natalie, and now three lovely grandchildren too.

He died 3 days after that anniversary in 2006. I continued my long career in nursing which has changed so much from those early years and in the last decade I focused on palliative care which was more in tune with my own values and beliefs on patient centred care. I retired last year as all the NHS changes finally wore me down!

I'm writing not to just tell you all this information but to let you know what a difference you have made to my life. You really cared, you made me feel like I was important, not just another NHS patient. You listened and believed in me. I don't often talk about that time to many people, but when I do I say how you made me feel safe and I believed that you wouldn't leave me – and you didn't. I left and never told you what a big impact you had on my life and that I knew I would never sink into those dark depths of depression again, I felt healed. That experience influenced every area of my life and work and the person I became.

Radical changes have taken place in mental care over the years but it wasn't just about the system, I was so fortunate to have had you as my Doctor. I don't know how difficult it was in those days to keep me as a patient when you moved hospitals, but you did and it made all the difference. I've never forgotten, it's just taken me a long time and before any more time passes, I just want to say a heartfelt 'Thank you, you saved my life'.

Best wishes

Sally Baynes

Sally Baynes (Davies)

3. Letter 2

15 June 2013

Dear Sally

Thank you so much for your candid and unsentimentally heartfelt letter.

I very quickly recalled your face and your spirit though, interestingly, I cannot remember your 'clinical' details, your 'history'. It is instructive, what we retain of one another.

I find your letter remarkable for the span of time you recall and the unaffected clarity and veracity of your account. I am deeply gratified and moved that the 'cuttings' I offered you so long ago were cherished, planted and nurtured by you and have steadily borne fruit, over a lifetime. In parallel it has been my conviction, over my working lifetime, that this kind of activity should often lie at the heart of what we do for one another. In these realms most damage and most healing is human.

It sounds to me as if your 'recovery' has gone far beyond the medically mapped realms of 'symptom relief' and 'good clinical outcome'. You indicate that most wondrous and humbling transformation: you have turned your painful burden into a compassionate and healing gift, for yourself and others. It seems that this has cascaded through your marriage to two generations of family, and beyond that to your many recipients

86

of palliative care nursing. All of this is heartening for me, too: our healing and nourishment of one another is often unobvious.

But there are shadows, too, where I also wish to join you. You refer to your 'patient-centred values and beliefs … being worn down', leading to your retirement (from the NHS). Likewise, your reference to 'radical changes in mental healthcare' making your own previous healing experiences most unlikely now. I resonate with this: such concerns are at the centre of my vocational life.

We are here different in our adjustment: you have expediently retired to your more accessible gratifications of family and grandchildren; I remain contentiously engaged with heroic obstinacy, possibly because I do not yet have grandchildren (though the social and biological machinery looks promising).

It seems that as we get older we find solace and peace in a few simple and timeless maxims: 'Counting our Blessings … Seeing what is there, not what is not …'. Simple to say, yet often so difficult to live by. It sounds as if you have managed a great deal.

Your letter has particular and intense value for you and I. But I think it has messages that are universally important, especially for healthcare workers. What you talk of lies before, behind and beyond all trainings, texts, systems, manuals, data and codes which now weary and alienate so many.

With suitable safeguards, could we publish these letters?

Whatever your reply I have found it deeply satisfying to have heard from you in this way: such communications give great difficulties even deeper meaning.

With warmest wishes
David Zigmond

Ω

(Private correspondence with an ex-patient, 2013 – with her consent for publication)

NHS Savings?

Abolish the Internal Market

The Internal Market is a failing experiment aiming to submit complex Welfare to monetarism and commerced industrialisation. Our earlier federal system addressed human and economic needs with much greater directness and honesty.

Recently, Sir David Nicholson, NHS Chief Executive, raised alarmed questions about how the NHS can possibly be paid for in the near future.

Throughout a working lifetime as a GP I have carefully watched many changes. I now have a pragmatic but retro-radical suggestion: we should abolish the entire Internal Market and thus such subordinate institutions and devices as the purchaser-provider split, autarkic and competing Trusts, payment by results and Commissioning. All of this may be well intended but is a failing experiment to apply commerce and Monetarism to complex welfare.

The human and economic costs of this defederalised system are very high. As fragmentation and boundaries increase, so do procedural, bureaucratic and financial complexity and delay. Competition, or its threat, decreases professional synergy and replaces it with expensively expedient tactics and presentations: glossy brochures, specious statistics, mistrustful feints, 'gaming' the systems and being guided more by technical legality than humanistic ethos. I have hundreds of examples documenting these, but rarely (if ever) discern clear benefits of defederalisation.

Here are two commonplace and recent examples. First: my locality GPs have cumulatively invested hundreds of hours tendering competitive plans for an Out of Hours Centre: this was a politically prescribed project of no real value: it evaporated without sense or trace. Second: at a mental-health centre I attended a dreary, droning, dead-eyed meeting where eight fractiously obedient practitioners discussed for half an hour a patient who none of them had ever met; in particular whether, or not, the referral was procedurally correct. Until recent times this would have been dealt with by a friendly five-minute phone call by an experienced practitioner with good sense and courtesy. Time and energy were then saved; helpful relationships fostered.

Such losses and follies may seem comically grotesque to an outsider: as an insider I know the enormity of the consequences: the costs to people as well as budgets – such is the maturing culture of corporatized and marketised Welfare.

The old, federal, 'Socialist' NHS did not have these problems. Yes, it had others but I think they were more honest and more soluble.

Ω

Published as a letter to *The Guardian*, 16 July 2013

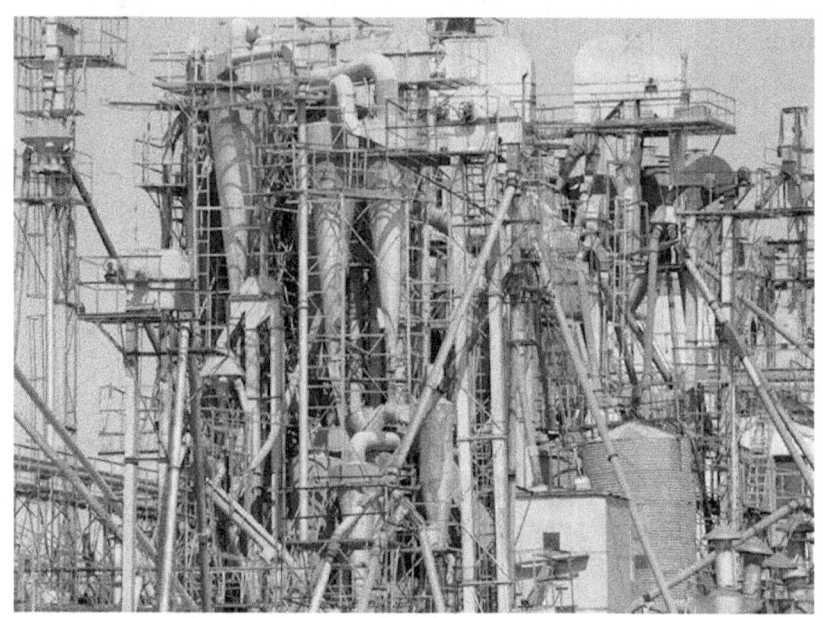

How Care Pathways obliterate Care

More industrial follies from the NHS

Overschematisation in complex welfare will usually yield results quite different from those intended.

Recently many seemed shocked by the malign metamorphosis of the Liverpool Care Pathway. For here we have an attempt to mass-produce and standardise compassionate palliative care for the terminally ill then contorting to a designed absence of care that combines shocking insensitivity, psychopathic expedience (hastening death to vacate usable bed-space) and chilling indifference to the suffering of the dying and their relatives. I am not shocked but wearily despondent: I work in a health service where 'progress' is increasingly defined by the displacement of the best, discriminating personal healthcare by didactic, 'expert-committee' generated systems which attempt to command quality by prescribing some kind of uniform plan. Industrialisation of dying sounds stark; it is. Most such schemes are doomed to very serious losses of personal connection and imaginative compassionate understanding. In any matters of human complexity institutional schemes and human understandings are often countervailed, unless we take great care.

The story of the Liverpool Care Pathway is like a Brothers Grimm fairy story even more unfit for children. It is an example of what can happen if we do not take that care. For the care of the dying is a poignant and delicate dance: each encounter requires unique responses of contact, utterances, understandings and technicalities. This is fine and fragile work that calls on any practitioner's capacities of empathic imagination quite as much as technical knowledge. It is the discriminating weaving of these that makes up the art of Medicine. With the characteristic follies and losses of our times we have largely crushed or displaced both the habitats and activities of such art in our healthcare in an attempt to get factory-like efficiency, compliance and uniformity.

Healing and palliation are complex interactions that arise from human kinship, not object-like management. Mind-sets and management modes from industry or commerce have very limited contributions to make to complex welfare. It is when their influence exceeds this that we have the toxic moral vacuum phenomena of Mid-Staffs or the Liverpool Care Pathway.

Ideas that seem easy in areas of great human complexity usually have a large and horrible price. As the philosopher Alfred North Whitehead said: 'seek simplicity, then always mistrust it'.

Ω

Published in *The Daily Telegraph*, 23 July 2013

The High Price
of Commodified Healthcare

Commerce, industrial manufacture and monetarism are seriously flawed bases for Welfare provision. This brief letter presents another snapshot of what is happening.

.

On one evening in the last week there were two separately channelled TV programmes addressing yet more apparent incompetence in NHS Healthcare. Each of the two programmes focused at opposite ends of a spectrum: the 111 Service for acute and short-term directive contact and then psychiatric services for the complexly distressed, for longer-term care. From this wide span of missed and miscommunications what common themes emerge?

The programmes' portrayals were consistent with my many decades' experience as an NHS doctor. What we are witnessing is the loss of a healthcare culture of personally invested connections and understandings. This has happened through attempts to emulate industrial manufacture and commercial trade. Before twenty years ago there was much good practice that was free of the current errors. For example, I was part of a GP out-of-hours rota which – together with our telephonists – provided a much more skilled, competent and personable service with little administrative clutter or expense. Likewise, when I worked as a psychiatrist I was able to offer personal continuity of care over many years with the commensurate containing, and healing effects: this was humanly rich yet financially economical. These lost patterns of healthcare extended beyond sensitive and sensible care for patients, they were – indirectly though substantially – sources of human nourishment and enlivenment for healthcarers too: the doctors I know may now be paid more, but they have less personal work satisfaction.

In complex human Welfare if employees do not really like their work they are unlikely to ever do it well, whatever the strictures and structures. A commercially or industrially modelled system becomes – perversely – humanly disconnected, then harmful and economically wasteful. The evidence for the failure of this approach is now ineluctable: it is a doomed project. We now need to largely dismantle these well intended but corrupting devices: autarkic and competing Trusts; commercial subcontracting; payment by results; hegemonic Goals and Targets, algorithms, Care Pathways and statistics-before-sense. We need to understand and reclaim the underlying motivational and vocational psychology of our work: why and how should we care for one another?

Our complex human bonds may then be better honoured.

Ω

Published in the *Guardian*, 7 August 2013

Psychiatry?

Everyone is right – but not for long

Psychiatry and physical medicine are often contiguous, sometimes continuous. This is subtle and precarious, for careless conflation can be harmful: we need vigilant discernment to prevent this.

.Will Self has done us all a service by provoking an interesting and telling correspondence ('Psychiatry, drugs and mental healthcare's future', (Guardian letters 8.8.13). What is demonstrated is that Psychiatry is like its erstwhile Rorschach (inkblot) projective tests: it can plausibly represent – even 'justify' – almost any of our fears, hopes, explanatory notions, preoccupations or prejudices. We can easily people it, too, with heroes and villains.

Yet if we heed certain distinctions we can avoid much confusion. For the territory and predicaments of psychiatry are often different from prevailing physical medicine. Psychiatry engages a protean realm of dis-ease, whereas much of medicine is more stably anchored to a solid world of disease. Dis-ease – our more undifferentiated human ailments – contains much that cannot be satisfactorily objectified or measured, as well as offering us endless puzzles of coexistent contradictions: these are due to the fact that our dis-ease is often a pre-verbal signalling system to ourselves and others that all is not well, that we are disequilibrated.

Both kinds of veterans – the Psychiatrist (Professor David Goldberg) and patient (Trish Oliver) – write with convincing sense of the massive blessings of psychiatric medication applied when dis-ease is so great that it is not just contiguous to, but seems continuous with, disease: this is 'major mental illness' and its designation is often problematic because this must rely mostly on human experience and judgement. Unlike physical medicine, attempts at objective testing of dis-ease often turn out to be more flawed than useful.

Most of us seeking help with substantial psychological distress do not have such major mental illness and require not didactically structured treatments but dialogically evocative forms of containment and healing. The former (treatments) may be accessible to standardisation, measurement and mass-production, the latter (healings) generally cannot.

Why is all this important? Because it leads to a predicament for current NHS Healthcare whose increasingly industrial, measurement-fuelled ethos will tend to favour the prescriptive treatment interventions appropriate to cure disease, rather than the imaginatively attuned healing encounters that may help us transcend dis-ease. This accounts for an increasing, sometimes tragic, discrepancy: as our technical treatments get better, our personal care gets lost. This is reflected in many of our recent grotesque headlines of institutional neglect and abuse. The over-prescription of psychoactive drugs is a commoner example, less dramatic but still important. Such skewed professional activity is often telling us that we are losing our best balance between the science of manipulation and the art of understanding. Yes, prescriptive and designatory psychiatry can provide great benefits, but its limits always need artful and humane discernment.

Good healthcare is a humanity guided by science. That humanity is an art and an ethos. Any wisdom we can bring to bear will be in the blending and balancing of these: the constitution of such wisdom must always extend beyond our formulae.

Ω

Letter to the *Guardian* 2013

NHS Healthchecks

more automation and less intelligence

The front-page story *NHS checks on over-40s condemned as 'useless'* (20 August) and subsequent letter (*Healthcheck checks*) can lead us to additional valuable insights into virtuously squandered resources and depleted staff morale in the NHS.

In the last two decades of my work as a GP my original role as a skilled, holistic, personal and family physician has been steadily displaced by imperatives to perform government-dictated generic and measurable procedures: a tick-box world for healthdroids. Goals and targets are now firmly welded to contractual payments to ensure conformity. Such obedience costs not just money and skilled time, but also the doctor's intelligent and imaginative discretion and – eventually – the experience and ability to make humane and sophisticated judgements.

The current overtreatment of 'high' blood pressure is a common example of such perverse consequences. GPs are now paid according to how many high blood pressures they can lower: *ergo* they are driven to treat a measurement, not the patient. This has created serious secondary problems, particularly among the frail-elderly whose prescriptively over-lowered (for them) blood pressure then often leads to dizziness, falls, collapse and serious injuries – always distressing, sometimes fatal.

What is getting lost in such mass-produced and formulaic testings and treatments are the erstwhile aspects of care that are intelligently discerning, personal and bespoke. This is not just injurious to patients and budgets – practitioners, too, become diminished, deskilled and demoralised. This happens because our sense of meaningful contact and satisfaction grows from the autonomous exercise of such skills: they comprise the now ailing heart and art of medical practice. Importantly, these are closely akin to compassion. The process of these losses may be insidious, but the consequences are more stark. We are already finding that the more we reduce vocational healthcarers to act as centrally-programmed healthdroids, the more horror healthcare headlines we have coming to us.

Ω

Letter to *The Times* (2013)

Re-establishing Personal Bonds and Understandings in NHS Care

Dear Jeremy Hunt
(Secretary of State for Health)

I am a veteran inner London single-handed GP with a working lifetime's interest in humanistic aspects of healthcare, its bonds and milieux.

I listened to your Conference speech last week and was heartened by some of your messages. Previous Health Secretaries have management-spoke almost entirely of strategies, goals and targets, new regulations and control and monitoring systems. But you, refreshingly, have expanded the language and thus the perspective. You talk of the culture of values, the nature of the personal bonds and attitudes, and how these constitute the personal care that so often lies behind and beyond generic treatments.

In the early 1970s I had several thoughtful and compassionate mentors who modelled and encouraged imaginative and person-centred care. As a young practitioner I was led to see how overly bio-mechanistic healthcare encounters impoverished both human understanding and therapeutic opportunities. My interest and concerns about this led to my long train of qualitative research and writing.

What I did not foresee in my early career was how much worse the human disconnections would become: I had not predicted the impact, for example, of computers, informatics or systems management. The benefits these bring are early, evident and alluring; the human price is more subtle and delayed.

In your speech you anchored your human-scale concern to practical proposals. One of these is of particular interest to me: your wish to restore and revitalise personal investment and continuity of care by reinstating GP Personal Lists for the elderly. I think this is salutary and pragmatic: a good foundation-stone. But I would like to see this re-found foundation widened to all age groups who have chronic, complex or protean difficulties – for it is this large healthcare territory that must have personal bonds and understandings to make therapeutic effects likely.

The current NHS has become better at technology-based treatments where cure is likely, but worse at humanity-based care where cure is unlikely or impossible. The former may parallel the optimism of youth; the latter is the fate of age. Care and cure often require different kinds of heart and mind-sets: this often requires a flexible, delicate weave – and this becomes impossible with systems that are over-systematised and over-prescriptive. I have explored and written about these problems for several decades. If you are interested I have attached a small sample of articles, with some brief notes of guidance at the end of this letter.

In your speech you described how much you had learned from your brief work engagements on the frontline of the NHS. Here is an invitation for a similar and deepening experience: come to my small inner-city General Practice and see my attempts at long-term, personal continuity of healthcare and the adversaries I have in institutions, politics and culture.

Meanwhile, thank you again for your humane and humanising contributions and plans: I hope you hold office long enough for them to grow securing roots.

Ω

Letter to Secretary of State for Health 2013

Loneliness in the Ailing Elderly: social and healthcare responses

Dear Jeremy Hunt

(Secretary of State for Health)

I heard of your comments recently. I am grateful that you are, again, broadening the language and thought from the systemic and managerial to include the humanistic and ethical.

I am a small-practice GP with decades of experience working long term with the kinds of problems you refer to: I would like to share some of my understandings.

I am sure you have far too much to read, but I am attaching two writings that are almost certainly different from your usual fare: they are personal narratives, written in a spirit of scientific enquiry, by a veteran frontline NHS doctor. The first, *The Psychoecology of Gladys Parlett* was written in 1988 and more prophetic than I intended. The second, *Five Executive Follies*, was written much more recently, for your predecessor, Andrew Lansley: it demonstrates and explains what has happened in the last two decades, since Gladys Parlett.

Of course, I shall be interested in any thoughtful response.

Ω

Letter to Secretary of State for Health 2013

Dr Frankenstein's Reprise

Industrialisation of personal healthcare: adverse effects of sequestered psychiatric in-patient services

Dear Dr Dratcu
(Consultant, In-patient Psychiatrist)

I am writing to you as a long-serving GP with a long but now increasingly consternated interest and experience in Mental Health. For many years I have accumulated both dismay from, and interest in, the riddle of our increasing personal disconnection in healthcare.

This letter is very long: this reflects not just the length of my observation and reflection, but also the protean complexity and multivalence of our tasks. Crucially, I believe it is our expedient oblivion and then short-circuiting of these essential subtleties that has led to many of our current errors. So this long missive is a small act of correction.

Yet though this letter may be unusually demanding, I hope it will be equally rewarding through attention. It is one of several I have written about areas of endangered or eroded personal care. For several years I have worked in a system where mental health services have become more humanly disconnected despite, apparently, good administrative coherence. Patients' experiences of psychiatric admissions provide clear examples of this.[1] The first part of this letter portrays the problems I encounter. Later I provide some little-discussed explanations and finally my ideas about the now very difficult restoration.

It is important that I first clarify that this letter is not a personal or professional criticism of you or any of your staff, though it is a critique of the system we are operating and the

107

culture it leads to. All the difficulties I describe may include, but extend far beyond, any individual practitioner. Though addressed to you, I am intending communication to be stimulated more widely.

*

First, let me tell you something of the background to this letter, and outline a more general view of our mutual problems: for many stymies we have in psychiatry, including your territory of acute admissions, are a constituent of this larger, ailing, puzzled jigsaw.

I am one of your local GPs. I am working in an NHS that is increasingly troubled by its own designs: by generating a more and more industrial-type system of rigidly boundaried fragments, defined by administratively categorised specialisations. The costs of the resulting human disconnection are high, but its subtlety also leads to expedient ignorance: over-systematised and depersonalised care has developed its own life and momentum: sleep-walking like a Frankenstein's Monster among the perplexed and vulnerable.

My concern about such healthcare misindustrialisation extends to all more pastoral areas of healthcare – those where the charismatic blessings of rapidly successful technology-based cure is unlikely: this constitutes much of mental health services and General Practice. I have been recently engaging with colleagues in these areas to stimulate creative debate. Amidst these wider concerns and efforts, the activities of sequestered In-Patient psychiatry continue to provide me regularly with graphic examples of the consequences of our healthcare follies. I have written previously to other mental health executives detailing some of my own and patients' experiences: I urge you to read them.[1]

Second, let me introduce myself. I am a veteran inner-city GP servicing a small practice in Bermondsey, your catchment area. In the first half of my career I did much qualitative research into healthcare human connections; what is therapeutic and what not, then why and how[2]. In more recent years this interest has become bound to my consternation that modern systems of diagnosis-centred management, in their attempt to confer precision and efficiency, are often overused and then become countertherapeutic.[3] This is obviously the reverse of what is intended, and further attempts to rectify the problems with similar methods will compound and compact the human disconnection. This is the corrosive paradox and conundrum we have generated throughout pastoral healthcare. This letter is part of my mission to widen and broaden thought and discussion.

*

Now I would like to return to our problems with acute psychiatric admissions.

I am currently caring for four patients who, in the last year, describe urgent in-patient psychiatric care at the Maudsley Hospital. Their individual stories converge with similar experiences of care: the emergent themes – of being cared for with impoverished personal understanding at times of intense vulnerability – are growing with our current accelerated systemisation.[4] Increasingly we have a system ill-equipped to offer havens of comfort, containment and personal understanding to enable natural processes of healing and recovery. Instead the overwhelmed, the dis-integrated, the disequilibrated – the acutely mentally ill – are hurried between relays of assessment and risk management teams: staff who usually have no prior or subsequent relationship with the patient.[5] All of this may make much sense to management. It does not for patients: for their inchoate agitations or utterances of distress – and then the personal understandings of meaning necessary to heal such breakdown – require a rapport involving personal continuity, patience and imagination: these are unlikely to survive on a conveyor-belt of short-term objectification. No kind of institutional or academic cleverness can substitute for personally evolved healing relationships.[6]

My argument here is separate from, though may be amplified by, those of scarcity of resources. There is, currently, a media conveyed interest in the lack of acute psychiatric beds.[7] This may also be a serious problem, but different to what I am addressing: my four patients were all 'lucky' to be promptly admitted to a local unit (The Maudsley Hospital). My questions here are not about funding or procurement, but the nature of such care. My view here is that in mental health it is often the failure or disruption of human bonds that sicken, and it is through certain kinds of careful human bonds and understandings that we heal.[8] Technical language and procedures may sometimes help such humanities, but rarely should they displace them.

*

I used to work both in, and with, psychiatric services that offered mental healthcare based on far greater personal continuity and thus understanding. Because of this, the previous services were more economically viable, too: a psychiatrist and his team who have developed a trusting, nuanced and personally understanding rapport with a patient are likely to have far greater therapeutic leverage and success than a rapid carousel of centrally-directed strangers, however well trained. But this is what we have now: the attempt to model such pastoral care on airports, surgical techniques or car factories leads to the abject disconnected 'care' described by my four patients.[9]

*

We cannot recreate the past, yet with intelligent analysis it has much to teach us. My early career experiences in now-vanished, better Mental Hospitals taught me much about the subtle values of longer-term personal bonds and understandings; of flexible and intelligent capacities for containment and asylum; and – conversely – the folly of sharp, excessive packaging – our expedient resort to rigid diagnoses and institutional care pathways. Such early lessons in thoughtful eclecticism guided and enriched my working lifetime, had decades of enthusiastic agreement among my peers and are supported by much historic documentation.[10] Sadly and importantly such lessons are increasingly lost or disregarded – this is one definition of cultural change.[11]

*

So, how can we transpose or transplant these lessons to our current situation? Here are some notions, caveats and suggestions to help us reconfigure mental health services in a way that restores my working maxim: Healthcare is a humanity guided by science. That humanity is an art and an ethos.

In Principle, we need to understand:

- How and why have we brought about these difficulties? I think much can be explained by a little discussed, but seminally important, shift of axioms in teaching and academia throughout mental healthcare. We have abandoned the previous equilibrium between phenomenology (a description and clustering of how things are, or appear) and semiotics (what things might mean).

- Phenomenology is more compatible with objective and scientific discourse and understanding. Semiotics is necessary for imaginative human understanding. So, phenomenology is more concerned with treatment: healing must draw largely from semiotics. A balance and easy exchange between the two is necessary for holism. Compassionate care is mostly impossible without holism.

- Partly due to the rise of computers, and then the seductive (often treacherous) opportunities to industrialise mental healthcare, there has been an increasingly demanding rhetoric to displace semiotics (an unmeasurable art) by phenomenology (a measurable proto-science, though often speciously so).

- Without intelligent discrimination this can easily lead to the follies of scientism: to services whose zealous attempts to make a science of manipulation is often at the expense of the art of individual understanding.
- We need to return to a personal continuity of care – sometimes over long periods. This can provide much better individual understanding and thence to humanly nuanced diagnosis and therapeutic influences. (The exceptions to this are always instructive and interesting.)
- Personal continuity of care is more an understanding and arrangement between consenting adults than a procedure decided by a Central Directorate.
- Nevertheless personal continuity – even when desired, optimal and unproblematic – must always be 'safety-netted' by background administrative and institutional continuity.
- Generally, when working well, personal continuity of care should be a pre-eminent and anchoring principle.

In Practice this means:

- Bringing back Consultant General Psychiatrists who would be responsible for running a team (these used to be called 'Firms' and typically consisted of the Consultant, one or two grades of trainees, a Psychiatric Social Worker, Community Psychiatric Nurse, Clinical Psychologist, Occupational Therapist and then his in-patient Ward Staff).[12]
- This Consultant Psychiatrist would be responsible for a geographical area and therefore would get to know families, streets, local myths and rumour, GPs, Social Workers, Health Visitors and District Nurses.[13]

- By having their own core-staff and in-patient Ward, the Psychiatrist, and the more long-serving members of the team, are then able to provide a much more personally-knowledged and engaged service.

- This locality-based, consultant-led team would provide the bulk of widely ranging psychiatric help for most patients who need it. The team would be responsible for the whole span of most patients' likely care: out-patient clinics, home visits (assessment, monitoring and therapeutic), day-patient and in-patient care.[14]

- For very refractory or unusual cases there would be tertiary centres to refer to.[15]

- This consultant and their team would then have the advantage of personal knowledge and understanding to make dextrous and effective decisions. For example, a psychiatrist with long experience of a patient is much more able to quickly and accurately evaluate a difficult and unstable situation and, say, admit the patient, or have the CPN visit regularly or get them an urgent Day Centre place, supervised by an OT. (This was much of my experience in the setting of large Mental Hospitals in early 1970s. Care was – comparatively – much more efficient, person-centred and seamlessly initiated and integrated. Holism was not explicitly talked about, but easily enacted. Staff conflict, tension and sickness was much less and morale much higher: people liked their work.)

- It is, therefore, not just patients who will benefit. Work satisfaction is much greater when personal investment is more valued and attachments last long enough to bear fruit that can be witnessed and savoured. Staff who derive warmth and satisfaction from their difficult tasks will work much better. This has benefits for both management and the economy.

- The dismantling of administrative barriers to more holistic and personal healthcare is needed throughout the NHS where pastoral care is elemental. For example, there are strong arguments for reinstating GP personal lists and hospital General Physicians.[16]

- The kind of Consultant Psychiatrist that I envision re-establishing resembles also the better old kind of General Practitioner in terms of their breadth of skill, accumulation of personal knowledge and long-term vernacular commitment. They would thus be more experienced, and thus older, on appointment. Their professional influences would derive as much from vocational education as hegemonic training.[17] This raises further issues about medical recruitment, training v education, and the design and finance of career structures: all need further complex analysis.[18]

*

I do hope you will read this letter with something of the thought and spirit that has gone into it. I certainly do not expect a long written reply, but I would like to begin some informal discussions. I am also inviting this from our Mental Healthcare Commissioners and Medical Director.

Notes and References:

[1] In this long letter I have not included a description or analysis of individual accounts that have provided me with grist and motivation. Similar stories can be found in earlier writings, which I have numerically referenced and are easily accessible via my Home Page. This applies also to related and cited healthcare themes.

Previous letters to senior colleagues might interest you. They are:

- *Eric: Another victim of Hypertrophic Obstructive Management Coagulopathy:* A letter to the Medical Director, South London and Maudsley NHS Trust (2012)

- *Bureaucratyrannohypoxia:* An open letter to Mental Health Services Director (2010)

The particular patients who talked with me of their depersonalised and unattuned in-patient experiences are willing to talk to you and other responsible healthcare workers.

[2] My interest in this has spanned a long career. See, for example:

- *Three Types of Encounter in the Healing Arts: Dialogue, Dialectic and Didacticism* (1987)

- *The Front Door of Psychotherapy: Aspects from General Medical Practice* (1989)

- *Why Would Anyone Use an Unproven Therapy? Treasures in the Mist* (2010)

[3] See, for example:

- *Idiomorphism: the Lost Continent. How diagnosis displaces personal understanding* (2011)

- *Institutional atrocities: The malign vacuum from industrialised healthcare* (2013)

[4] *Continuity of Care: Of course, but whose? A Sleight of Slogans: Letter to Family Doctor Association* (2012)

[5] *If you want good personal healthcare, see a Vet. Caveats for holistic healthcare Part II* (2012)

[6] *Sense and Sensibility: The danger of Specialisms to holistic, psychological care* (2011)

[7] Dr Martin Baggaley recently talked to the media about the loss of psychiatric in-patient beds. He was there talking of *quantity*: my

concerns here are *qualitative* and different, though they may be parallel.

8 *Mother, Magic or Medicine? The Psychology of the Placebo* (1984)

Thirty years ago this article expressed a kind of imaginative, yet disciplined, *intersubjective* analysis often pursued by thoughtful practitioners. This kind of thought has become nearly extinct in the last twenty years. In my view this is largely due to our indiscriminate use of electronic informatics. This has generated an unwise and uncompromising rhetoric of *objectification*, whose language is data. Unmindfully unleashed, such data have a similar relationship to human imagination and relationships as swarms of locusts have to human habitats and crops – see *Words and Numbers: Servants or Masters? Caveats for holistic healthcare Part 1* (2012).

9 I documented this change in culture, and its human casualties in Psychiatry: *Love's Labour's Lost. The pursuit of The Plan and the eclipse of the personal* (2010)

10 I have many documents to itemise and date these changes. Two of them I have contextualised in:

- *Language is not just data: it is a custodian of our humanity* (2013)
- *Physis: healing, growth and the hub of personal continuity of care A thirty-nine (39) year delayed follow-up correspondence with Sally* (2013)

11 *Institutional atrocities: The malign vacuum from industrialised healthcare* (2013)

12 My earliest experiences in Psychiatry – in an old Victorian Mental Hospital in the early 1970s – provided an excellent (comparatively) personal service of this kind. Its positive influence has been indelible for me. See *Psychiatry: Love's Labour's Lost. The pursuit of The Plan and the eclipse of the personal* (2010)

13 The conception of the old general psychiatric team could be redesigned. Obviously they would not operate from a large Mental Hospital. Smaller, more numerous In-Patient units would be close to Day Centres, Out-Patients etc, ideally within easy walking distance. Geographical proximity and easy personal contact with colleagues lead to much better colleagueial understanding and relationships – see *Eric: Another victim of Hypertrophic Obstructive Management Coagulopathy* (2012).

14 These reincarnated General Psychiatrists would function much like the better GPs of this earlier period: they guide and care for many different kinds of patients over long periods, will often delegate to known colleagues but retain an overarching interest, personal knowledge and responsibility.

This kind of sense of caring containment was mostly more therapeutic for patients: work satisfaction for the professionals was commensurate with this.

15 This worked well in the 1970s. Only a small fraction of more puzzling and refractory cases would be sent to a tertiary centre (eg for Severe and Uncontained Psychosis, Eating Disorder or for long-term Psychotherapy). This is paralleled elsewhere in the NHS: see note 16.

16 See my examples at the end of *Five Executive Follies: How commodification imperils compassion in personal healthcare* (2011)

There is a parallel argument to reinstate the erstwhile kind of General Physician who would provide the vast bulk of hospital-based secondary medical care. They (as before) would only refer on a small fraction of more complex work. Currently, older people are often under multiple medical specialists, each for a fairly common condition. Very often patients cannot name the speciality, even less the specialist: there are all kinds of losses here – of personal bonds and understandings that are essential to comfort and healing; to speedy, accurate professional judgements that come from personal familiarity; of efficiency that comes from uncomplex administration; of efficiency that comes from good work satisfactions from satisfying personal bonds.

General Practice, since the abolition of Personal Lists and the accretion and demise of small Practices, has very similar problems.

17 Consultants many years ago were usually less formally trained but more informally educated. They were older and thus had longer and wider experience. This may have been less neatly compact for managers but produced many unsystematic blessings.

See *No Country for Old Men: The Rise of Managerialism and the New Cultural Vacuum* (2009)

[18] There is a welter of problems in all this. What are the alternatives to the current severe academic meritocracy to gateway Medical Schools? How can we best encourage education (learning by enquiry) without losing the hard essentials of training (assurance by instruction)? If (as I would argue) Psychiatric Consultants should have longer and wider prior experience of healthcare and life, how would we encourage this without loss, to them, of money or motivation?

Ω

Letter to the Medical Director, In-patient Psychiatry, Maudsley Hospital, South London, 2014

Post-scripted appendix: Early reply from Dr Dratcu

6 November 2013

Dear Dr Zigmond

It was a pleasure talking to you on the telephone. I am honoured that you have decided to share your thoughts with me. I am also very pleased to see that you have such wide and longstanding interest in, and understanding of, the ever changing framework within which mental health services operate, and the implications of this to our patients.

You have written a very detailed document and I apologise for not addressing it point by point. May I nonetheless start by saying that many of the concerns you have raised are exactly the same that I and a significant numbers of my colleagues frequently entertain about developments in mental healthcare provision within the NHS. We are all aware of the fragmentation of mental health services in recent years and its pitfalls. We are also aware of the challenges that many management-driven approaches may engender in our interaction with our patients. In an age where IT and databases increasingly encompass everything we do, there is indeed a risk that all this may culminate in what you describe as "increasing personal disconnection and industrialisation of healthcare".

These are clearly broad issues that go far beyond mental healthcare alone, and for which we are unlikely to have easy answers. With your permission, and as we discussed on the telephone, the best course of action for me at the moment is to divulge your message to my colleagues.

Kind regards

Luiz Dratcu

Dr Luiz Dratcu, MD PhD FRCPsych
Consultant Psychiatrist, Maudsley Hospital

Qualifications
may be less than useful

D. Stewart's letter ('Qualifications aren't everything', Independent, 2 November 2013) conveys much robust sense and sensibility. Our world of Welfare services is increasingly strangled and obstructed by excessive and rigid technical requirements. As a veteran GP in the NHS I have seen how damaging this has been. NHS healthcarers are now more highly trained and qualified than ever, but this is often at the expense of humane and vocational spirit. Our technical treatments are undoubtedly better, but our personal and pastoral care is often worse. The now-frequent headlines of healthcare-horrors are tips of icebergs: under the surface we will find much more.

Yes, technical procedures need specific training and qualifications. But the complex needs we have in our care and guidance of one another requires much more, and that more is often very different. Compassionate interest and imagination are subtle and natural fruits. They may be induced, encouraged and modelled, but then cannot be directly or didactically instructed or assessed.

More worrying, an attempt to technicalise personal care and understanding will often destroy them. More of something 'good' is sometimes worse.

$$\Omega$$

Letter to *The Independent* 2013

We need an Appointment with Dr Finlay

A recent article by Stephen Moss ('Pills, bills and bellyaches: a peek behind the scenes at a GP surgery', *The Guardian*, 3/11/13) is a vivid Hogarthian portrait of a frontline of our current NHS.

As a long-serving inner-city GP there is much I can endorse, amplify or dispute. One strand is of interest and illuminates much else. Health Secretary Jeremy Hunt is reported as pressuring *simultaneously* for a return to a traditional 'family doctor' ethos (which I strongly support) and an instant, Skyping, emailing, extended hours service (which I find inimical). It seems clear to me that one service cannot do both, and that an emphasis on the latter will destroy the former. Personally sensitive and imaginative care requires certain kinds of understanding, and these can come only from attentive human contacts and bonds.

The article then notions the various types of GP arrangements: consortia, businesses, partnerships and polyclinics. These are considered as options for future service delivery. What is not returned to is the *small* practice with its strong vocational ethos and long vernacular roots. The better examples of these could, and did, provide much better human contact, understanding and containment than the current large-scale alternatives. Small practices may not have advantages of economies of scale but they can save much – in both human and economic terms – by restoring subtle and important human connections and understandings.

When my small, single-handed practice closes it will be dissolved into something much larger and less personally sentient and responsive. In my old age it is most unlikely that I will receive the kind of care I have been able to offer for so long. I will want it.

Ω

Published on *BMJ blog*, 2013

Dementia is not only (or even) a Disease: it is a Signal of our Community Cohesion

In recent weeks there has been much written about dementia, including articles by your correspondent Max Pemberton (*Dementia sufferers must have specialist care*, 2/12/13) and the Health Secretary (*Why I truly believe this generation can be the one to overcome dementia*, 29/11/13). While I certainly agree with their analysis and concern about the size and seriousness of the problem, my understanding of the nature of the problem is importantly different.

Both write of dementia as if it can be tackled head on – 'to beat dementia' – as we have done substantially with HIV and some cancers. But there are crucial (if unwelcome) differences: much dementia is a natural correlate of advanced age and not necessarily a pathological variation. Partly due to medical technology and partly due to social mobility we are living longer, but then have prolonged and slow declines in relative social isolation. This is now the usual and embedding matrix of dementia.

Medical technology currently has little to directly offer to most such cases of dementia. What helps much more is responsive, sensitive and imaginative guidance and containment. This is pastoral healthcare and welfare: twenty years ago the better GPs, district nurses and social workers were able to do this much better than now. Personal continuity of care – one of the best contributions to such welfare – has been made almost extinct by the successive devices of managerial systematisation and industrialisation of healthcare.

No, we do not need a massive new tranche of dementia clinics, consultants and brain-scanners: we need to retrieve the kind of social workers, GPs and general hospital physicians who can build personal relationships with patients, their

123

families and communities – often over many years. No, we cannot 'beat dementia', and substantially may never do so. But we can, and should, offer professionally wise and compassionate counsel and containment to people we can get to know, understand and care about. This is good, personal, pastoral medical care of a traditional kind. Its retrieval sounds less inspiring and glamorous than 'beating dementia', but it is more realistic and thus achievable.

Ω

Letter publ. in the *Daily Telegraph*, Dec. 2013

Thank Goodness we now have business-sense to safeguard our Welfare

Commercially injected Welfare Services are managing a magical amalgam: combining venal corporate capitalism with leaden, officious, State bureaucracy. Here is one tiny example: we can expect much more.

*

We are living in worryingly ingenious times. Example: I have just paid fifty pounds to a large profit-making Corporation, subcontracted by the local council, for them to issue me with a Certificate, in order for them to collect my non-clinical refuse. They know that my clinical waste is disposed of by another (non-commercial) agency. Because I am a GP I am posed certain questions to certify my good citizenship and thus guarantee public safety: I must answer that I will not put such things as used dressings, sharp surgical instruments, excised body parts, unwanted organs, bodily fluids or dead babies in the general waste. They will not collect my waste without their (my) Certificate, which I can only purchase from them. They do not check the accuracy of my answers.

This is a brilliant conflation of venal, opportunistic, corporate capitalism and laden, vacuous, officious bureaucracy: it exemplifies much that is most specious, profligate and foolish in our commercially injected welfare services. Whatever happened to medical office effluent before such corporate vanguards were there to protect us, and the Certificates issued to 'prove' it?

Ω

Published in the *Independent*, 27 January 2014

Failure of Personal Continuity of Care in Mental Health Services

The high cost to patient and practitioner welfare and the health economy

Dear Mr Lamb
(Minister for Care, Dep. of Health)

I am a long-serving GP with much additional experience working alongside and within mental health services.

Recently, I heard you talking on the Today programme (6.5.14). You were responding to concerns about our services' difficulty in providing good quality response and containment for the acutely mentally distressed.

It is a common view that our major problems are primarily due to inadequate resources, training or management. This may be partly true. But I think there is a more important though more subtle problem: the progressive loss of personal continuity of care throughout the NHS. I have watched this with growing alarm for many years: my long view motivates this long letter.

Our loss of more personal types of understanding and care is not easy to understand. It is a kind of 'collateral damage': its evolution is insidious, complex and paradoxical. For example, it can seem incontestably beneficial to always increase the schematic and 'objective' in our healthcare: but pastoral healthcare (ie our human responses to all those problems that do not have quick and definitive fixes) is chimeric, and these measures can then easily displace or destroy its many kinds of meaningful but fragile bonds: our relationships. This often happens without much awareness: we later awake and are shocked by their absence. Our current mental health services – both acute and chronic – are replete with such paradoxes: of how density of schematic management is often inversely proportional to therapeutic meaning for the patient. Every working day I do what I can to rectify many exigencies from this. I have forged for myself and my patients a precarious respite to do this: I have battled to retain a stable small practice. So, for many years I have still, with some difficulty, provided a kind of countervailant personal perspective and continuity: this kind of vantage is now very rare.

*

Throughout pastoral healthcare our best therapeutic engagements come from personal understandings. And these must come from growing bonds, each of which – like each individual – has both commonality and uniqueness. By not heeding this we are creating many more problems. For such personal bonds fare poorly in services that are complexly remote, highly managed, sharply boundaried and fragmented. The human casualties from this make for some shocking stories: I have witnessed and documented many. Yet these industrial kinds of services design do have a better place: for example, they are much more compatible with clearly anatomised physical disease – though even there we are finding serious problems emerging; even the most biomechanical needs some carefully bespoke care.

*

Pastoral and biomechanical healthcare are countervailant, yet complementary and synergistic. They are apparently opposite, yet we must combine them in innumerable ways. The art of evoking this synergy is a good definition of holism. But such holistic practice is now ailing and imperilled, for recent schematised healthcare reforms have often deracinated our personal bases of pastoral care. Inevitably, we then lose our more holistic views and understandings. In General Practice and Psychiatry – my areas of work – the losses are most clear and grievous.

*

How can we repersonalise our now humanly enucleated pastoral care? In the wide spectrum of the NHS the remedial principles converge, but the applications vary. Yet whatever the variation, we need to retain this seminal anchoring principle: personal continuity of care. For it is primarily from the development of personal attachment, affection and understanding that healing and palliation can take root. What we are now witnessing is serial examples of how all of this disintegrates in large, fragmented organisations that tend to standardised procedures. So, what specifically can we do to restore NHS Psychiatric Services? Here, in outline, are my summarised suggestions and bridging explanations:

- We need to bring back Consultant general psychiatrist-led 'Firms' (this is an old term for consultant-led teams).
- These teams would be locality-based and would take the vast majority of the wide variety of more severe mental and behavioural distress.
- The Consultant, with necessary deputies, would take overall responsibility for the complete cycle of mental healthcare from first contact to (provisional) discharge. (The bracketed word is necessarily important, if unwelcome.)
- The Consultant's Firm would have three major 'limbs': for Out-Patient consultations, for Home Visiting and for In-Patient Care. These three limbs would have some cross-flow and overlapping of staff (eg a patient is likely to be seen by the same practitioner(s) in a clinic, a ward, a Day-Centre, or at home).
- Most importantly, patients could move dextrously between different aspects or phases of care (Out-Patient, Day-Care, In-Patient and Home-based) with the kind of speedy and intelligent sensitivity that can come from personal continuity.

- Such personal continuity confers personal and economic benefits. Lengthy, cumbersome-yet-blind, bureaucratic assessments, procedures and documents become unnecessary. This cuts administrative burdens, costs, errors and frustrations drastically. Patients, generally, feel more contained, understood and comforted by people with whom they have an enduring bond. Staff have the slow, deep 'parental' satisfactions of seeing things through – the therapeutic effects of personal continuity are not confined to the patient!

- Obviously the Consultant Psychiatrist needs help with all this. The typical Firm would also contain trainee and deputy psychiatrists, psychologists, nurses, occupational therapists and social workers. As in well-functioning families there is, generally, easy and apt overlap and interchangability of roles, though some important areas of sequestration.

- Most therapeutic encounters would thus be delivered and monitored within the Firm. When other skills are required (eg for more intensive psychotherapy, Day-Centres, or more unusual or refractory cases) the Consultant would (with the help of their other professional staff) make tertiary referrals to more specialised units.

- The Consultant's Firm would therefore be looking after patients in Clinics, In-Patient Units, Day Centres and at home. Ideally all of these are easily commutable from one another.

- Much psychiatric work is with people whose complaints fluctuate over many years. A relapse can be much more humanely and effectively responded to and contained by staff who already have developed bonds of personal knowledge and understanding.

- Likewise In-Patient discharges are likely to be far less problematic if a patient continues to receive guidance and support by the same team that tended them in times of greater distress.

- Of course, personal continuity of care is never complete or perfectible. It is a value and a guiding principle. In the untidy and buffeted real world all kinds of compromises are inevitable or advisable.
- The General Psychiatrists' work would thus resort to a wider base of more 'parental' personal responsibility. Their professional development and appointment would depend, as in previous eras, more on length and breadth of experience and education. This is in contrast to what we have now: a pressure to successive, modular, technical-type trainings to accelerate earliest promotion. (This itself raises many questions about the selection and process of medical trainings v education.)

*

What do I base these ideas on, and why do I think they will work?

From the early 1970s I worked in Psychiatry for many years. In that time we were able to provide much better personal continuity and quality of care than is generally available now. This more personally continuous care was not only more meaningful and satisfying for staff and patients, it was also more efficient: our decisions had greater speed, sensitivity and appositeness. This was less expensive.

Almost all my cohorts from that period take this view. They are, however, at retirement age and most are too beleaguered or weary to argue: their resonance with these views now exceeds their public articulation.

If you are interested in reading about particular scenarios and patient-situations, together with my expanded analysis of the problems and our responses, then I would like you to read my letters and submissions to senior managers and clinicians of our Mental Health Services. They are available via my Home Page.

In addition I have collected hundreds of relevant NHS documents over many years. Each one provides salutary and graphic evidence for these ideas.

I want to end this letter with another paradox and an ensuing invitation. The paradox: I prefer pithy, live dialogue to prolix, abstract documents. The invitation: my Practice is ten minutes of easy Underground travel from (or to) Westminster. If you, or one of your deputies, wish to discuss these matters, it would please me greatly.

Ω

Letter to the Minister of State for Care, Dep. of Health 2014

Renationalisation
of the Rail Services?
Why not, instead, start with the NHS?

Recently the media has told us that the Labour Party is considering a long-journeyed return: back to the nationalisation of rail services. Some claim this will offer better long-term value, efficiency and safety.

Many would welcome this, but there is a puzzling anomaly: why do we not, instead, start with the NHS? For, surely, the contentious market principles of competitive commissioning are better suited to human transport than human healthcare. This is an important distinction, and our failure to recognise the difference between the mechanical and the human has led to a new tranche of serious NHS problems.

For twenty-five years we have had successive governments push through legislation to extend the control, reach and leverage of the NHS Internal Market. Yet almost all senior practitioners with long prior experience agree about the human and economic cost consequent to our depersonalised fragmentation of the NHS. This has been engineered by such commercialising devices as competitive commissioning and autarkic NHS Trusts. Cumulatively they have been highly destructive to both the quality of continuity of care, and the morale and trust of staff. The Royal Colleges have consistently taken this view. From my own long-serving GP practice I have hundreds of documented cases to illustrate these organisational follies.

Personal knowledge and continuity of care may matter little in the carriage of passengers. It matters a great deal in the care of the complex human interweavings of the ailing body, mind and spirit. The NHS Internal Market is like Communism: a failed ideological experiment. Such ideologies may start with some aspirational ideas of merit, but these must always be diluted and titrated. For they are only partial and conditional truths, and our failure to heed the difference between guidance and dominance has led to our failed massive social experiments.

Yes, a reconstituted national British Rail could possibly offer us greater economy, choice and comfort. What an intelligently refederalised NHS would offer us would be much more. Here is another anomaly: why now do we hear no substantial challenge to the existence of the Internal Market from our usually glad-to-be-contentious opposition politicians?

Ω

Publ. by Open Democracy 2014

The Author

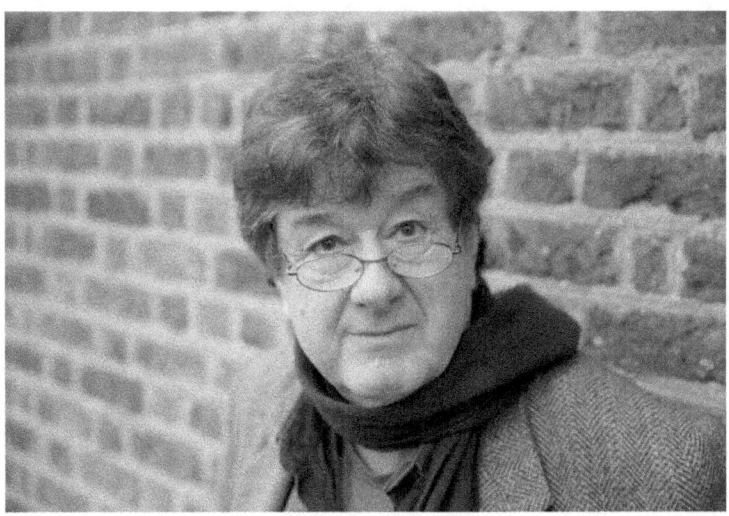

David Zigmond initially trained in Medicine in the 1960s. For several decades he has worked in the NHS as a small-practice GP, and as a large hospital psychiatrist and psychotherapist. Alongside these he has maintained a practice as a private psychotherapist. From these long tenures he has explored the nature and importance of relationships, imagination and personal meaning throughout healthcare. These have fuelled and guided his view and practice of holistic medicine. His long-spanned teaching and writing have been committed to develop and secure these values.

He helped launch the British Holistic Medical Association in the 1980s and has remained active in developing this approach. This book contains many of his contributions.

Other Books on Health
by New Gnosis Publications

Wilberg, Peter *The Illness is the Cure - 2nd extended edition: an introduction to Life Medicine and Life Doctoring - a new existential approach to illness,* 2014

Wilberg, Peter *from Psychosomatics to Soma-Semiotics: Felt Sense and the Sensed Body in Medicine and Psychotherapy,* 2010

Wilberg, Peter *Being and Listening: Counselling, Psychoanalysis and the Ontology of Listening,*2013

Wilberg, Peter *Heidegger, Medicine and 'Scientific Method': The Unheeded Message of the Zollikon Seminars,* 2012

Wilberg, Peter *Meditation and Mental Health: an introduction to Awareness Based Cognitive Therapy,* 2010

Wilberg, Peter *The Therapist As Listener: Martin Heidegger And The Missing Dimension Of Counselling And Psychotherapy Training* 2008

Zigmond, David *If you want good personal healthcare – See a Vet Industrialised Humanity: Why and how should we care for one another?* (Complete collection, 716 p) 2015

Zigmond, David *The Psycho-ecology of Gladys Parlett – Hidden personal meanings in healthcare* (If you want good personal healthcare – See a Vet, Volume 1) 2015

Zigmond, David *From Family to Factory – Lost personal meaning in healthcare* (If you want good personal healthcare – See a Vet, Volume 2) 2015